# Words Of And Praise

"*The Do's and Don'ts of Low Blood Sugar* was chosen among the top best lay medical books of 1988 - 1989 because it covers a subject of potential interest to public library patrons in a responsible, easily understood way. ... A worthwhile edition to a public library collection."
*American Library Journal*

"*The Do's and Don'ts of Low Blood Sugar* has been endorsed in our programs. Only those books that are felt to be truly outstanding selections are incorporated into our programming. It's always a personal pleasure to encounter and recommend good, conscientious work to our audience."
James A. Cox, Editor-in-Chief
The Midwest Book Review
Oregon, Wisconsin

"You've done a superb job after years of both personal and intellectual research on this topic. Thank you for helping so many people who will benefit from your experiences and clear writing."
Jeffrey S. Bland, Ph.D.
Gig Harbor, Washington

"This is a great book. So easy and so practical. Just right for the hypoglycemic who seems to fade after concentrating for 10 minutes. You are writing for all those with a short attention span."
Lendon H. Smith, M.D.
Portland, Oregon

"Congratulations on a great little book that really brings the whole question of low blood sugar into an easy to read, understandable form. You certainly answer every conceivable question that a patient is likely to ask and I wish you every success."
Robert Buist, Ph.D.
Sydney, Australia

"I appreciate having received your book. The focus for me was chapter ten, in which you discussed the approach to a positive attitude. I love the way you formulated your concepts and am happy for you that the book is in print."
Leonard A. Wisneski, M.D., F.A.C.P.
Bethesda, Maryland

"My first suggestion to a hypoglycemic patient is to read your book. Education and understanding of hypoglycemia, or LBS, is probably the single most important thing that one can do to deal with this condition and your book is a great place to start."
Douglas M. Baird, D.O., P.A.
Palm Beach Gardens, Florida

"Thank you for sending me a copy of your book. The time and effort which you put into it really has paid off. You have an excellent, well written and informative book. I will be sure to show this to my many patients who are suffering with hypoglycemia."
Irving Karten, M.D., F.A.C.O.G.
Hollywood, Florida

"Your latest book on low blood sugar is FANTASTIC! You have successfully distilled the essence of the subject for those that suffer from the often misdiagnosed and misunderstood condition of hypoglycemia. The information on diet, vitamins and exercise could easily be followed by anyone who is seeking health or wants to maintain their health."
Leo B. Stouder, B.S., D.C., D.N.B.C.E.
Hollywood, Florida

"As I began to read your book, I couldn't help but feel that I was reading my own story with all the frustrations and fears that you experienced. I would also like to say thanks for all your time and effort you put forth in getting this book published and the Hypoglycemia Foundation started."
Madison, Wisconsin

"The book was a tremendous lift to my spirits and renewed my courage to keep up the pace on the road to recovery. I wish that every person who has hypoglycemia or is suffering the symptoms and doesn't know the cause could read this book. It is a great support!"
Selma, North Carolina

"I believe your book, *The Do's and Don'ts of Low Blood Sugar*, could be the most helpful thing a newly-diagnosed hypoglycemic could read. Its simplicity of style makes it an excellent first choice. How I wish it had been available to me in 1980."
Del City, Oklahoma

"I have just finished reading your book, *The Do's and Don'ts of Low Blood Sugar*, which I picked up at the library. It is the most informative information I have found to date."
East Lyme, Connecticut

"My doctor has informed me that I am "borderline diabetic" and he has recommended that I read the book entitled, *The Do's and Don'ts of Low Blood Sugar*.
Summerland Key, Florida

"I just read *The Do's and Don'ts of Low Blood Sugar* by Roberta Ruggiero from the library and feel hopeful that there is a lot more information out there. The book was terrific!!"
Roswell, Georgia

"...I have scoured bookstores and health food stores and every place else I could think of for information. I was quite discouraged until yesterday when I went to the library. I found a copy of your *Do's and Don'ts of Low Blood Sugar*. I was thrilled with all of the information you included in this book. From my own experience I know how much work must have been involved in gathering it. I finally feel like my husband and I will be able to get a handle on our situation and keep his condition in check."
Houston, Texas

"Your book *The Do's and Don'ts of Low Blood Sugar* was a life saver. After more than 15 years I have finally found my cure: a simple diet!"
Poland, Ohio

"I have read it and found it very helpful. The way it is written makes it very readable and clear and very interesting because it is written from a personal point of view."
Southport, Merseyside (England)

"I read your book recently, *The Do's and Don'ts of Low Blood Sugar*. I wish I had found it before I did all my technical reading. The book made me cry. It also made me feel as if I was being hugged and comforted by a dear friend. You wrote so well about all the things I've been trying to explain to my family as well as to my doctor."
Kew Garden Hills, New York

"I want to thank you for opening up a new world for me."
Ft. Lauderdale, Florida

"It was like looking in a mirror to read your book."
Ft. Lauderdale, Florida

"Since I read your book - it has saved my life - literally."
Paris, Kentucky

"I am a 38 year-old hypoglycemic, recently diagnosed and I cannot thank you enough, Roberta Ruggiero. It was because of your book - *The Do's and Don'ts of Low Blood Sugar*, that I was able to recognize myself as a hypoglycemic, and I asked my doctor to test me. He, although skeptical, agreed, and to my delight my hypoglycemia was confirmed beyond a doubt. This singular diagnosis has finally explained away a lifetime of symptoms, physical and emotional, and has helped me and those nearest to me understand that it was not nor is not my "nature" to be miserable, touchy, disagreeable, negative, etc, etc, but it is only a very controllable disorder which causes me to become that way."
Niagara Falls, New York

"Thank you for changing my life!"
Holland, Michigan

# THE DO'S AND DON'TS OF LOW BLOOD SUGAR

## AN EVERYDAY GUIDE TO HYPOGLYCEMIA

*by*

*ROBERTA RUGGIERO*

*President of the Hypoglycemia Support Foundation, Inc.*

Library of Congress Cataloging-in-Publication Data

Ruggiero, Roberta, 1942-
    The Do's and Don'ts of Low Blood Sugar.

    Bibliography: p.
    1. Hypoglycemia—Popular works.    I. Title.
RC662.2.R84    1989    616.4'66                                    88-45456
ISBN 0-8119-0791-0

The information in this book is not intended as medical advice. Its intention is solely informational and educational. It is assumed that the reader will condult a medical or health professional should the need for one be warranted.

For information:
Lifetime Books, Inc.
2131 Hollywood Boulevard
Hollywood, Florida 33020

Library of Congress Catalog Card No. 88-045465
International Standard Book No. 0-8119-0791-0


3 4 5 6 7 8 9 0

Dedicated . . .

To every hypoglycemic—particularly those who have been mistakenly told that their symptoms were "all in their head."

The Hypoglycemia Research Foundation, Inc.
was founded
on June 6, 1980
but was renamed
The Hypoglycemia Support Foundation, Inc.
on December 13, 1991.

# Table Of Contents

*The order or length of each topic does not reflect its importance or value. Only when they are all incorporated to preserve and prevent illness can a patient truly reap rewards.*

*Please Note: The terms hypoglycemia and low blood sugar are used interchangeably throughout the book, but have the same meaning.*

# Acknowledgements

The best part about writing this hook is remembering everyone who played a role in its creation. They not only influenced my work, but also my life.

Gratitude goes to the hypoglycemics who have shared their story with me; every professional, medical or otherwise, who said yes to an interview; the Board of Directors, the Board of Advisors, and all of the members of the HSF, as well as the volunteers who gave so generously of themselves.

I would like to give special attention to the following: Douglas M. Baird, D.O., Hewitt Bruce, Ph.D., Emanuel Cheraskin, M.D., D.M.D., Arthur Ecoff, D.O., James W. Johnson, D.C., the late Robert S. Mendelsohn, M.D., and Stephen J. Schoenthaler, Ph.D. Each and every one of you was instrumental in my growth. As mentors, teachers, healers, and most of all friends, your directions, reassurances and confidences gave me the courage to continue working toward my dreams.

I would like to give special thanks to: Toni Crabtree, Lois Frimet, Shirley S. Lorenzani, Ph.D., Theresa Mantovani, Karen McCoy, Marie Provenzano, and Lorna Walker Ph.D. —on a professional, personal and spiritual level, each of you combined your strength and support to spur me on during my most difficult times.

Special thanks go to Harvey M. Ross, M.D. for his valuable suggestions and for writing the preface; David Kohn for using his editing expertise to polish this manuscript; and the Staff at Lifetime Books, Inc., who gave this book love and tender care from the moment it was placed in their hands.

And, a very special thanks to my children, Renée and Anthony, and my husband, Tony. Their unconditional love, patience and understanding, gave me the freedom to do my work and to make this book a reality.

# Preface

I have treated people with hypoglycemia since the late 1960s. I've learned by listening to my patients about the multiple frustrations that they experience, starting from the time they first begin to recognize something is wrong to the numerous visits to doctors over the years. Then, too, there are the frustrations experienced in their professional and personal lives right through to the confusion in treatments and difficulty in adhering to a program once it is outlined. Through her experience, first as a patient, then as an advisor who reaches out to thousands of others to help them through their difficult times, Roberta Ruggiero has learned to help people recognize this illness, find professional help and, finally, help to comply with the programs suggested for the treatment of hypoglycemia.

In *The Do's and Don'ts of Hypoglycemia*, Roberta shares with her readers the rich knowledge of her own experience. She is able to guide, teach and support those with this problem; a problem that is, more often than not, overlooked or even scoffed at by the majority of those in the medical profession.

If you have, or even suspect that you or someone you know has hypoglycemia, this is the book for you. By following the "do's and don'ts," those with hypoglycemia will be able to reduce and even eliminate their symptoms, and start on the road to a more fulfilling life.

Harvey M. Ross, M.D.
Los Angeles, California

# Introduction To Second Edition
## Of
# The Do's And Don'ts
# Of Low Blood Sugar

I wrote the first edition of *The Do's and Don'ts of Low Blood Sugar* with a tremendous amount of fear and self-doubt. Here I was writing a medical book with no medical degree and writing about a condition the medical community labelled a non-disease. Even those who did recognize its existence, still called hypoglycemia the most confusing, complicated, misunderstood and misdiagnosed condition of the 20th Century.

So, why did I write it? And even more importantly...why am I back again...five years later, writing a revised edition?

It is because of you, the readers. You have written to me, cried on my shoulder, begged for more support groups, more information, more research, more concern and more caring.

From big cities like Los Angeles, to little-known towns like Soddy, Tennessee; from Canada to Great Britain; from Alaska to Ireland, letters have poured in. Many of these are still enshrined in my heart and soul.

The letters, the phone calls, the outreached hands...that's why I'm back again.

I've added more do's and don'ts to most chapters. Additionally, I've added two new chapters: one Health and Beauty: You Can't Have One Without The Other and another Letters

From Our Mailbag, in which I share some of the letters I have received. They are too heart-wrenching and too important to keep to myself.

I've consulted with the experts once again: the mentors, teachers and advisors who have guided me and the Hypoglycemia Support Foundation for the past twelve years. As always, they have responded. Each of these individuals has given freely of his/her time and expertise. Their love, commitment and understanding have enabled the HSF to continue...to succeed...and to grow beyond my wildest expectations.

However, I must confess there were times when I wanted to give up. The road has been rocky, the work hard and lonely. At times, so frustrating that I would say..."That's it!...No more!..I quit!" And then, as always, someone would call and say..."Wow, your book saved my life"!...or..."Your information saved my marriage"...or..." I thought I was alone, but now I feel as though I have an understanding friend."

All of this was confirmation...confirmation of what I have known all these years. My personal experiences with hypoglycemia, years of mis-diagnosis, ECT treatments (Electroconvulsive Shock Therapy) which took years of therapy to overcome and the problems of trying to run an organization with no financial assistance were tests...tests to challenge my strength, courage, determination and persistence. Slowly, but surely, my grueling challenges became glorious triumphs. I was vindicated.

Believe me, at times I feel like I'm the selfish one, because in helping others, I'm helping myself. I've grown emotionally, intellectually, mentally and spiritually. Isn't that what life is all about, living life to its fullest...not just existing! I've been blessed a hundredfold. The people I have met, been privileged to work with, and the people I've been able to open up to...to share with, to confide in, to laugh and cry with...my family, friends, brothers and sisters of this incredible universe...you are among my greatest blessings.

# Introduction

If you think you may be going crazy; if you have thoughts of suicide; if you're constantly exhausted, anxious and depressed; if you go for weeks without a decent night's sleep; if your personality changes like the flip of a coin; if a counter full of munchies doesn't satisfy your sweet tooth; and if your doctor thinks you must be a hypochondriac because medical tests don't show anything physically wrong with you -- don't despair, there's hope!

You may not need a psychiatrist, or even pain pills, tranquilizers or anti-depressants. Surprisingly, a simple DIET may relieve your symptoms!

This condition, which is confusing, complicated, misunderstood and too often misdiagnosed, is hypoglycemia, or low blood sugar. According to leading medical authorities, it affects one-half of all Americans, including celebrities Burt Reynolds and Merv Griffin. It is most frightening because most people who have it, don't know it. Often, the myriad collection of symptoms are blamed on other causes.

I know because I've been there. I suffered with hypoglycemia for ten years. Numerous medical specialists, dozens of tests, thousands of pills, and even the administration of electroconvulsive shock therapy (ECT), did nothing to eliminate my symptoms.

A simple glucose tolerance test (GTT), proper diet and strong determination finally led me down the road to recovery. Unfortunately, it took years. If only I had had the knowledge that lies between the covers of this book, my journey would not have been so traumatic.

To help others avoid what I experienced, to bring to them the causes and effects of hypoglycemia, and to give support, encouragement and enlightenment to those suffering this insidious disease, I formed the Hypoglycemia Support Foundation Inc. (HSF) on June 6, 1980.

Through the HSF, I have had the opportunity to speak with thousands of "searching" hypoglycemics. They all are looking for the best doctor, diet, book or miracle cure. They are asking the questions that I once asked: What should I eat? Should I take vitamins? Should I exercise? Why isn't my diet working? Why doesn't my family understand? Can I ever eat out again? More serious questions commonly asked are: Why doesn't my doctor recognize hypoglycemia? He says it's just a "fad" disease. Is the glucose tolerance test necessary? How can I find a physician sympathetic to a hypoglycemic's needs? The list is endless, and so, sometimes, is the pain.

During this time, as I was trying to educate hypoglycemics, they in turn, educated me. They told me what they needed and wanted and, above all, what they were not getting. I learned of their pitfalls, anxieties and fears. Coupled with my own feelings, everyone I encountered seemed to respond with the same universal phrase, "If only I had known . . ."

There are many good books out on the subject of hypoglycemia. However, when I insisted that a patient get a book to read about his or her condition, I began to realize that, although this was valuable advice, most of the people, unfortunately, were in the first stages of hypoglycemia, a time when the mind is confused, the body is weak and concentration is difficult.

When I found myself repeating the same guidelines over and over again, I realized that these patients first needed simple, easy-to-read, concise and comprehensible guidelines to help them handle their condition. They needed a prerequisite, a book to read BEFORE all the other books on hypoglycemia. They needed a book with specific do's and don'ts written in layperson's vocabulary before grasping for medical definitions and explanations.

This is what I hope to achieve with *The Do's and Don'ts of Low Blood Sugar.* Use it as a key to education, interweave it with commitment and then, love yourself enough to take the final step -- application! Are you ready?

# 1

## *Letters From Our Mailbag*

**W**hy devote a chapter strictly to letters that I have received? The answer is quite simple. I am hoping the following letters will have some of the same effect on you as they had on me. I am hoping that the connection that was formed, the bond that was cemented... and the feeling that flowed between the writer and me... will be passed on to you, my reader. I want you to benefit by gaining inspiration from the challenges and triumphs experienced by other hypoglycemics and learn from their mistakes and their successes.

Together, let's shed more light on hypoglycemia which it needs if the sting is to removed from it's tail. The following letters will speak for themselves.

Dear Roberta:

THANK YOU, THANK YOU, THANK YOU!
The information you have been kind enough to share with me
has been the key link enabling me to return to a normal life.

Several months ago, I began growing faint and was, on
about half a dozen occasions, taken to the emergency room of
a local hospital. In every instance, I was told there was nothing wrong and that I was probably just hyperventilating. After
consulting several doctors without any success at all, I was
properly diagnosed by a local physician who recommended a
glucose tolerance test. Once it was determined that I had
hypoglycemia, I was referred to the Cleveland Clinic for dietary
planning.

The staff at the Cleveland Clinic were enormously
helpful but referred me to you and your organization for additional help. The materials you have supplied me have helped
me understand my problem and do what is necessary to return
to a normal life. I am saddened by my own experience with
the many doctors who were unable to determine what was
wrong with me. I am frightened for the many thousands of
patients throughout the country with similar problems who are
no doubt experiencing the same kind of difficulty with their
diagnosis. I hope for their sake that they will be as fortunate as
I was to be directed to you and your wonderful, caring organization.

Please let me know if there is anything I can ever do to
repay the enormous debt I owe to you.

Sincerely,
Fort Lauderdale, Florida

Dear Roberta,

Thank you...Since I read your book (it saved my life, literally) about 3 years ago, I've been on again, and off again the diet. I usually go back on my diet after a very bad episode, such as my pancreas killing me, or I start blacking out again.

Only those who've had this devastating illness can understand how one understanding person who writes a little book (you & your book) can save so many people from unnecessary reactions such as suicide.

I wrote to you once before several years ago crying my eyeballs out. Finally, after my entire life and several doctors telling me everything but, Hypoglycemia, it was good to know I was not nuts.

Thank You!
Paris, Kentucky


Dear Roberta,

I have just finished reading your wonderful book for the second time and I can't tell you how much it helped me. It's such a terrible disease to have, it was the most trying time of my whole life, I thought I was going insane for sure. It started out for me about seven months ago, I got out of bed one morning and started to have a panic attack, (which I had never experienced one in my life), and thought I was having a heart attack. My husband was at work and my children, ages 7 and 3, were still asleep, so I called my neighbor and she took me to the hospital and they told me it was my nerves and gave me a shot and sent me home. After that I kept having panic attacks, anxiety, and severe depression, so I went to my doctor and he gave me nerve pills and said that it had to be something in my subconscious that was triggering all of my symptoms. I just knew that it was something physical because I started to develop a lot of other symptoms after that and I would go back to my doctor and tell him that the pills weren't helping and about the other symptoms I was getting and he almost acted mad because I wouldn't take his word for it. I feel that God really had his hand in all of this because my family and friends were all praying for me and my neighbor (who took me to the hospital), her daughter has hypoglycemia and she thought that I could have it, because she had the same symptoms that I was having. So, I went back to my doctor again and I asked him if he thought I could have low blood sugar and he sort of laughed and said that most people who have panic attacks think they have that or else a brain tumor. I feel that he just agreed to give me a 5 hour GTT to humor me and I think it really offended him because I was right and he was wrong. My blood sugar level went down to 46 in the third hour of my test, when I called his office to get the results, he didn't even talk to me on the phone, his receptionist told me I had low blood sugar and made an appointment for me to see a dietician at the hospital. She, (the dietician), was very helpful and she even said she couldn't understand why doctors don't recognize and check people for hypoglycemia more often. . . .Three days later I called a different doctor and made an appointment and had all of my medical records transferred over to him. Well, I am so happy that I switched doctors, my new doctor took a complete family history and said that I am a prime candidate for hypoglycemia with having diabetes in my family and I also had diabetes with my first pregnancy. He felt that 46 on my GTT was no doubt low and he's following up on everything, too. He wants to see me every six months to check for diabetes and to see how I am doing.

I am so thankful that I didn't have to suffer a real long time, like you or some of the other poor people in your book, before I found out what was wrong. I am thankful too, that now I have a lot more good days than bad ones. It is so nice to have a doctor who is understanding and recognizes how dreadful it is to have this disease. I just don't understand why all doctors don't recognize hypoglycemia, it is really a shame to think that there are so many people out there who are having terrible mental and physical problems and they probably have low blood sugar and might never know that they can feel better just by following a diet!

Thank you for writing your book and sharing your story with so many others, I'm sure it has been very helpful to everyone who reads it and also, thank you for forming HSF.

Thank-you
Saginaw, Michigan


Dear Ms. Ruggiero:

I recently came across your book *The Do's and Don'ts of Low Blood Sugar* and would very much appreciate any information (nutritional or otherwise) you may have regarding Hypoglycemia. As I began to read your book, I couldn't help but feel that I was reading my own story with all the frustrations and fears that you experienced. I would also like to say thanks for all your time and effort you put forth in getting this book published and the Hypoglycemia Foundation started.

After 10 years of being treated as a manic depressive, 20 electroconvulsive shock therapy (ECT) treatments, and being placed on every anti-psychotic and anti-depressant medication on the market, I was finally rediagnosed as hypoglycemic. Since I have changed my diet accordingly, I feel 100% better the majority of the time. ...

Thank you for your time and attention you have given this letter. I have suffered quite extensively these last 15 years and have no desire to repeat this experience! Therefore, any information that you can provide me with will be most helpful.

Sincerely,
Madison, Wisconsin

Mrs. Ruggiero,

I was so happy to have found your book, *The Do's and Don'ts of Low Blood Sugar*. I'm 26 and have known for several years that I had hypoglycemia but knew little more than to stop eating sugar. I followed the 'sacred diet' faithfully for years but never seemed to get much better. When I asked about what to do I was given another copy of that diet, patted on the back and was told that I would be just fine if I left the sugar alone. When I called the office confused and wilted, I was told to get a candy bar and that would bring my sugar up and I would be fine. The confusion mounted. That was when I decided that I would find out on my own what I should do. So, I hit the libraries. That is where I found your book. I felt like you had written the book after spending a few months watching me. It really was nice to finally know that I was dealing with something conquerable.

Your book marks the beginning of my quest for information on this quiet culprit who sets up camp in the corner of your life and robs you of your senses. Even though I still find myself in unexplainable tears or wrapped in a blanket in 90 degree weather, I finally feel hope. I feel sure that God has His hand in this matter. Thank you for writing and sharing your experiences and knowledge.

God Bless You,
Milford, Michigan


Dear Mrs. Ruggiero,

I can't tell you how enlightening your book, *Do's & Don'ts of Low Blood Sugar*, was for me. My daughter was diagnosed with hypoglycemia in August of '91. We had been having problems with our daughter since around puberty, she is now 17. Her grades were slipping, she was always in a strange mood and her temper seemed to flash out of the blue. She just didn't seem like a happy adolescent. My daughter has always been independent and a handful but I thought these changes were just part of puberty. When we would get on her about school she would tell us she was studying but found it hard to remember what she read. My husband and I would just shake our heads and say she just wasn't putting enough effort into her work. We even had her tested for LD problems but the test proved negative. By the time she entered high school she was having headaches, first thing in the morning, which I figured could be a migraine but she never liked school, was doing poorly, so I figured most times it was a ruse to get out of school. Then we started with dizziness. By the time we reached August of '91 she was complaining of almost passing out. At this point we took her to the doctor. She had the Glucose Tolerance Test (over 5 hours) and was diagnosed. We were given a diet, told this was common in teens and she would probably outgrow the problem. It seemed no big deal. The doctor said to keep on the diet for 3 months then start reintroducing foods - looking for the dizziness as a guide. Also artificial sweeteners were fine. Natural fruit juices were also acceptable, no restricted amounts.

By this time I had talked my husband into Family Counseling. It seemed what I thought was a family was disintegrating around me. I was an emotional mess. It never dawned on me to read up on her hypoglycemia. I could only concentrate on one thing at a time and counseling was it.

Counseling seemed to be helping out but we still had periods of uneven behavior. I had read an article in the paper about behavior problems with hypoglycemic kids and asked the doctor if this was   true. He said, "No way, don't give her that handle to use." I believed him. Why? I can't answer that, not even now. After a year - almost all of the foods had been reintroduced. She has reported no dizziness but erratic behavior, even worse than before. Our counselor had her evaluated by a psychiatrist who diagnosed a long term depression. When she was arrested for battery last week I called our counselor and asked for his help. His first thought was a reevaluation. His supervisor overruled this and they had a staff meeting instead. In on this meeting was the supervisor, our counselor, the psychiatrist and a psychologist. They concluded that she had a "Personality Disorder" and I had to accept her as is. We were also on our own and they wished us good luck.

Two days after this verdict my daughter brought home your book. (My daughter works at a library.) I can't even describe how I felt as I read this book. The pain, the guilt, the unbelief that I could be unaware of this for so long. That I had put my daughter through hell because I didn't do my job as a mother. I tried calling the counselor - I didn't even know if he told the staff that my daughter has hypoglycemia. We had told him when we first started the sessions. He was honest with us. He told us he knew nothing about it, we explained what we knew from the doctor and promptly forgot about it.

I don't know how to pull this together. I can't let this diagnosis stand as is if the hypoglycemia wasn't taken into account, which I feel it wasn't. I know that my daughter will not miraculously turn into Mary Poppins but if LBS accounts for even a small percentage of her problems I feel it should be reevaluated.

I need advise. I've set this trap by my own ignorance but I don't want my daughter to pay for my mistakes.

Sincerely,
Mokena, Illinois

Dear Mrs. Ruggiero,

Thank you for writing your book, *The Do's and Don'ts of Low Blood Sugar*.

In 1980 I was diagnosed as hypoglycemic by an alert and caring physician. Bless him. Even though I was not subjected to many of the horrors most hypoglycemics experience when they first realize 'something' is wrong I well remember the feeling of having been transported to some twilight zone where nothing made sense as I struggled to understand my condition. My own experience convinced me it takes two people, a knowledgeable doctor and an informed patient, to manage this condition. In my attempts to understand hypoglycemia, what it is and how to treat it, I read most of the literature available to the average person. Given my belief that education is essential to the hypoglycemic it is still my policy to read everything available on the subject. I believe your book, *The Do's and Don'ts of Low Blood Sugar*, could be the most helpful thing a newly-diagnosed hypoglycemic could read. Its simplicity of style makes it an excellent first choice. How I wish it had been available to me in 1980.

Sincerely
Del City, Oklahoma

Dear Sir/Madam,

When I asked the consultant endocrinologist who diagnosed Reactive Hypoglycemia, for some information, he replied "It's a well documented condition, look it up".

My G.P. (family doctor) and any of the Casualty Officers who have seen me as an emergency have never heard of the condition, and do not want to believe it exists. The population of this country is so small that the margin between a minority and a freak is very narrow. Information is difficult to find. A literature search in a university library has turned up a list of textbooks written in the seventies and early eighties. The science of nutrition seems to have developed since publication of these texts. I am trying to find any articles or published papers of a more recent vintage on hypoglycemia/ neuroglycopenia.

I am groping around in the dark here, trying to find a workable regime by trial and error. If you can suggest where I might find up to date information, it would be a great help.

Yours faithfully,
Bray, Co. Wicklow, Ireland

Dear Sirs,

I was thrilled to find Roberta Ruggiero's book, *The Do's and Don't of Low Blood Sugar*, and find out about your organization! My symptoms of hypoglycemia began in 1984 after the birth of my daughter. I knew there was nothing physically wrong with me so I thought I must have been going crazy. My mood changes were too frequent and drastic to be normal. I knew we could not afford a psychiatrist so I made an effort to cope with the problems on my own. It may have been a blessing in disguise, however, because I was not given tranquilizers and other drugs and therapy about which I've heard horror stories. My symptoms grew to include sudden hunger, weakness, dizziness, nervousness, fatigue, confusion, depression, etc. I suffered for four and a half years until finally a sympathetic doctor agreed to give me a glucose tolerance test. It was then that my suspicions were confirmed and I discovered that I was definitely hypoglycemic.

It has been almost a year since my GTT and I am finally beginning to feel that I am making progress. My doctor, sympathetic though he was, gave me the wrong advice about my diet telling me that I needed more sugar. As a result I spent about five months eating the wrong things, and my symptoms got much worse instead of better. A friend recognized what was happening to me and put me on the right track. I am doing much better now, but am still not as well as I would like to be.

That is the reason I was so glad to find Mrs. Ruggiero's book. I was beginning to lose ground and get depressed about my condition again, feeling that it was a never-ending battle. The book was a tremendous lift to my spirits and renewed my courage to keep up the pace on the road to recovery. I wish that every person who has hypoglycemia or is suffering the symptoms and doesn't know the cause could read this book. It is a great support!

Thank you so much for such a helpful book and for letting me share my story with you, though I'm sure you've heard it hundreds of times from others! Thank you for all you are doing to help others with hypoglycemia!

Yours truly,
Selma, North Carolina

Dear Roberta,

I want to thank you for opening up a new world for me. Coming into the Hypoglycemia Support Foundation is a major step in my journey, and I am now proud to be a member.

God Bless
Ft. Lauderdale, Florida

Dear Ms. Ruggiero:

I just read your above mentioned book which I enjoyed very much. I have been suffering from depression for the past 30 years. I have seen numerous top doctors around the world and not one doctor had suggested that I take the glucose tolerance test. ...

Regards,
Montreal, Quebec

Dear Mrs. Ruggiero:

I read your book recently The *Do's and Don'ts of Low Blood Sugar*. I wish I had found it before I did all my technical reading. The book made me cry. It also made me feel as if I was being hugged and comforted by a dear friend. You wrote so well about all the things I've been trying to explain to my family as well as to my doctor. ...

Sincerely,
Kew Garden Hills, New York

Dear Roberta,

Thank you so much for your call. I can't tell you how honored I felt. Since I got over the shock that my condition was "nutritional" and not "mental", I always felt that there was something I should be doing so that others would not needlessly have to go through what I went through. You took that step and I hope that I can contribute to help spread the word! ...

Sincerely,
Topeka, Kansas

Gentlemen,

... As a physician in general practice now sensitive to hypoglycemia as a real diagnostic entity who routinely screens it, and, as a husband trying to help my wife normalize her life, I am requesting your help. ...

Thank You,

Ft. Worth, Texas

To Whom It May Concern:

Please help me!  Tell me what I can eat that will make me feel better.  Tell me how much to eat and when to eat it.  I need recipes that don't call for deboned chicken breasts or artificial sweeteners.  I need recipes, menus, some reason for wanting to eat this stuff—and a diet plan that my family can eat too without killing off the whole bunch of us!

Eau Claire, Wisconsin

Dear Roberta Ruggiero,

Perhaps what I really need is to not feel so damn alone in dealing with my situation.

Thanks Again,
Spring, Texas

# My Personal Experiences

There was no turning back. After years of trying to hide my deep secret, I was now sharing it with what seemed to be the world. Tallahassee's "Capitol News" quoted me verbatim on May 9, 1978. It stated that Roberta Ruggiero, a former shock treatment patient from Cooper City, called the therapy "barbaric," saying she would "rather die than go through electric shock again."

The trail from private mental patient to public notoriety started out rather innocently. After my first child was born in 1961, I went into a deep depression. I couldn't stop crying. I had heard of postpartum depression, but mine was a deluge of tears that did not end. My family physician kept assuring me that my reaction was normal, and that it would go away. When it didn't, he introduced me to my first tranquilizer -- Valium.

Then the headaches started. The pain was there in the morning when I woke up, and persisted through my waking hours, and sometimes through the night. The pounding got so intense it felt as though my heart was actually throbbing inside my head. I was then given pills to reduce the pain.

I began having difficulty sleeping at night. Trying to get up in the morning was even more of a task. I became tired and weak. Cooking and cleaning the house, which I had always enjoyed, became a dreaded chore. I began to skip breakfast, hardly eat lunch and just nibble at dinner, if I had the energy to cook.

In 1963, I gave birth to my second child. All of my previous symptoms were compounded by dizzy spells and blurred vision. My nerves, needless to say, were hopelessly frazzled. My hands and feet were constantly cold to the point of feeling frostbitten. Even with medication, my symptoms got progressively worse. My doctor put me in the hospital for a multitude of tests: laboratory, X-rays, spinal taps and electroencephalogram. All the tests came out negative. There was nothing physically wrong with me. I began to think beyond a doubt that I was going crazy. I withdrew into a shell, avoiding contact with my family and friends because I was too embarrassed and ashamed to face them.

It was at this point that my doctor recommended psychotherapy. I spent several months with the first psychiatrist. He thought that perhaps the strain of getting married at an early age (18) and having two children 16 months apart, were the major contributing factors to my illness.

Maybe a "contributing factor," but not THE reason. When the psychiatrist put me on heavy doses of anti-depressants, I went to psychiatrist number two. It was a repeat performance.

My pain and symptoms were being drowned with strong medication pills to calm me down, pills to help me sleep, pills to relieve pain that was the order of the day. But since medication and therapy were not enough to relieve the symptoms, much less stabilize them, a third psychiatrist suggested electroconvulsive shock therapy, known simply as shock treatments! By this time, I was desperate and would have tried anything. The year was 1969, and in addition to all of my physical and emotional pain, I began to feel guilty about what I was putting my husband through. I agreed to go away and have what I believed was the "cure" -- my last hope.

I was wrong. I had not anticipated that my hospital room would have bars on the windows and doors. I didn't know that my clothing, wedding ring and "Miraculous Medal" would be taken away. And even more frightening were the screams, stares and glassy eyes of the patients who had already received treatments. I'll never forget the cot and its leather straps that bound my hands and feet, the electrodes that were put on my temples, and the rubber gag inserted in my mouth. The memories haunt me to this day.

After my first treatment, while I still had some faculties intact, I begged to go home, or at least speak to my husband. If he knew what I was going through, he would stop them. They said no. I had signed the papers for a series of electric shock treatments, and that's what I was going to get.

I had eight treatments in eleven days. The results were horrifying. I am thankful I don't remember all of them. I do remember feeling like I was in a state of limbo. My mind was functioning, but was not in coordination with the rest of my body. Despair, shame, guilt and thoughts of suicide remained. Approximately ten months later, I reluctantly agreed to another series of treatments, but this time on an out-patient basis. It was at the end of this series, that I swore I would rather die than ever be subjected to electric shock treatments again. The physical pain was nothing compared to the feelings of isolation, embarrassment and humiliation they caused.

With no solution in sight, we took the advice of our family physician who suggested that a change of scenery or a move to another state might offer some relief. It would be like a fresh start. Therefore, when my husband had an opportunity to move to Florida, we didn't hesitate.

Our move was exciting. I began to feel a little better. The pain in my head began to go away. Just having the sun shine every day seemed to promise a future where none had existed for so long. Then, suddenly, it happened again. This time, though, a new symptom assailed me. I began having fainting spells. I agreed to go for one last medical consultation. Dr. Arthur Ecoff, an osteopathic physician, examined me, reviewed my records and suggested a glu-cose tolerance test. I had never had this test before and was skeptical that a diagnosis could be reached. At this point, I would have settled for any diagnosis!

The GTT was taken and I was told I had a severe case of functional hypoglycemia. I was ecstatic! At last, I had a diagnosis, a name and a cure! But, to both my bewilder-ment and surprise, instead of a bottle of pills, injections or vitamins, I was given a DIET! Good-bye Yankee Doodles, Devil Dogs, hot fudge sundaes and apple pie. Hello chicken, fish, fresh vegetables, whole grains and fruits. I thought, "This is going to be a cinch."

Unfortunately, what I hoped would be an "overnight" remedy turned out to take several years of sorting through a mass of confusing and complicated information. Due to the unfamiliarity with the stages of recuperation, the controversy surrounding its treatment, and nonacceptance from many in the medical community, I found myself with the feeling of being the only person in the world suffering from this baffling disease.

Eventually, success did come, but alleviating my symptoms was a long and slow process. It would have been quicker if only I had understood the importance of individualizing my diet, the necessity for vitamins and exercise, and the role a positive attitude plays in the healing process. Above all, if there were other hypoglycemics to lend support and encouragement, the road back to health would not have been so rocky. Faith, patience, determination and the boundless love of my family were the cornerstones to my recovery.

Consequently, I didn't hesitate for a moment when I came across an article in The *Miami Herald* appealing to anyone who had experienced devastating effects of electric shock treatments. A committee for patients' rights was lobbying in Tallahassee and, after listening to my story, was eager to have me testify before the state legislature on behalf of mental patients. My hope was to convince the lawmakers to put severe restrictions on the use of ECT and, better yet, give the glucose tolerance test before its administration.

Little did I know that my life would never be the same. My story appeared in newspapers and on radio stations. I was immediately inundated with phone calls and mail from all over the state.

Letters, like the following, became all too familiar.

"Please send information. I had undiagnosed hypoglycemia for 23 years, and during that time, I ran the whole gamut -- depression, weight gain, weight loss, anxiety, psychiatric therapy and institutionalization—until the proper diagnosis was reached. The glucose tolerance test revealed that I had a blood sugar level of 35! Since that time, I am like a new person. I follow the proper diet, enjoy life and have no apprehension about blacking out without notice."

"I was ecstatic to see your article. My case was diagnosed approximately four months ago by my chiropractor. My internist had written me off as either psychotic or a hypochondriac, or both."

This feedback was the inspiration for my decision to start speaking to both hypoglycemics and members of our community.

When I couldn't handle the flood of letters and phone calls, and when I realized I needed medical and professional guidance, the idea to form a support group became a reality.

And so, the formation of the Hypoglycemia Research Foundation, Inc., became official on June 6, 1980. I am proud to say that I believe that no other organization has accomplished so much with so little. When I say "little," I refer to practically no money, secretarial services, office equipment and supplies, private phone or office space. How did we survive? Through positive people, positive thoughts, endless hours of hard work, dedication and prayer -- plenty of prayer.

With no advertising, other than the few articles about the foundation that have appeared sporadically throughout the past eight years, we have developed a mailing list of more than 2,500 people from across the United States. Without asking, we have been placed on the referral lists of several local hospitals and organizations. We hold monthly meetings at which medical or professional speakers share their knowledge about hypoglycemia, whether it is from a medical, nutritional, psychological or holistic point of view. We don't advocate or endorse any particular person, product or test. We simply make the facts available

The HSF has participated in health fairs and seminars. I personally questioned more than 600 high school students as to their emotional health. I shouldn't have been surprised because I had already read the statistics, but I found an alarming number of these students to be depressed and unhappy. One student said, "I feel like a keg of dynamite ready to explode." Overweight students were on water fasts or getting diet pills from their doctors! Far too many were skipping breakfast, and even lunch, and living on candy and soda from vending machines. Among the 600 students, the main complaint was fatigue. Shouldn't this information be telling us something?

My greatest personal accomplishment was being coordinator of a research project studying the correlation between diet and behavior in juvenile delinquents. It was under the direction of Stephen J. Schoenthaler, Ph.D., a criminologist from California State College in Turlock, California. With the help and guidance of Douglas M. Baird, D.O., a physician in North Palm Beach and then an active board member of the HRF, the project took place at *The Starting Place* in Hollywood, Florida, with 35 juvenile delinquents.

We tested them physically, psychologically, nutritionally and chemically. The results, though not conclusive due to the lack of a placebo control group, are published in a book entitled *Nutrition and Brain Function* (Craiger Press, Basle, Switzerland, 1987). Future research for control studies are absolutely necessary in this area.

Finally, there is this book. It is the core of all that I have learned in the last ten years. I wanted to share it in the hope of sparing some of you from the crippling effects of hypoglycemia. It is my sincere hope that I succeed.

**3**

# Definition of Hypoglycemia

I 've read and re-read the definition of hypoglycemia at least a hundred times. I've been asked repeatedly, what is hypoglycemia, and, in turn, have asked the leading authorities in the field of preventive and nutritional medicine. Their answers, although similar, are varied. Some are more technical than others. One thing is for certain — the definition of hypoglycemia can be as diversified and complex as the condition itself, or as simple and easy as some of the steps to control it.

In simple layman's language, hypoglycemia is the body's inability to properly handle the large amounts of sugar that the average American consumes today. It's an overload of sugar, alcohol, caffeine, tobacco and stress.

In medical terms, hypoglycemia is defined in relation to its cause. Functional hypoglycemia, the kind we are addressing here, is the oversecretion of insulin by the pancreas in response to a rapid rise in blood sugar or "glucose."

All carbohydrates (vegetables, fruits and grains, as well as simple table sugar), are broken down into simple sugars by the process of digestion. This sugar enters the blood stream as glucose and our level of blood sugar rises. The pancreas then secretes a hormone known as insulin into the blood in order to bring the glucose down to normal levels.

In hypoglycemia, the pancreas sends out too much insulin and the blood sugar plummets below the level necessary to maintain well-being.

Since all the cells of the body, especially the brain cells, use glucose for fuel, a blood glucose level that is too low starves the cells of needed fuel, causing both physical and emotional symptoms.

Some of the symptoms of hypoglycemia are:

*Fatigue, insomnia, mental confusion, nervousness, mood swings, faintness, headaches, depression, phobias, heart palpitations, craving for sweets, cold hands and feet, forgetfulness, dizziness, blurred vision, inner trembling, outbursts of temper, sudden hunger, allergies and cying spells.*

After reading a list like this, one can see why hypoglycemia can be misunderstood and easily misdiagnosed. Don't be alarmed if you read other books that I recommend and see that the list is, in fact, even longer. Don't be confused and frightened when you read other definitions that range from a paragraph to several pages in length.

For the beginner, it is important that you first recognize that most often hypoglycemia is the result of a diet high in sugar, alcohol, caffeine and tobacco.

Before going any further, look at your dietary habits and/or any addictive traits. Start adding up the sodas, coffee, cakes and cigarettes you consume in one day. Keep track of how many meals you miss. Are you under a tremendous amount of stress with your spouse, children, boss, etc. . . ? All of these circumstances can give birth to a case of low blood sugar that can plague you for the rest of your life. Don't take your body for granted. Neglect it, and you'll pay a high price. Take care of it, and low blood sugar becomes an inconvenience that you can manage by yourself.

# _Is There A Doctor Out There?_

T he phone rang and I didn't want to answer it. I was going to be late for an appointment 20 minutes away. Reluctantly, I picked up the receiver and a woman's voice said, "Is this the Hypoglycemia Support Foundation?"

"Yes. May I help you?" I asked. She proceeded to tell me her story. It was one that I had heard hundreds of times before, but the tone of her voice was more despondent.

Usually, I can listen attentively, but this time my mind was on my appointment. "Please give me your name and address, and I'll send you some literature."

But the frail voice continued to speak "Please, please

help me. I'm begging you -- find me a doctor immediately. I'm anxious and depressed. I can't sleep at night and I can't get up in the morning. I have an incredible craving for sweets. I read an article on hypoglycemia and believe that could be my problem. When I asked my present physician to give me a glucose tolerance test, he refused. He prescribed Valium. Please, before I get hooked on tranquilizers, I want to see a doctor who will listen to me."

I shuddered, and my heart sank. An overwhelming feeling of helplessness set in. I forgot about my appointment and listened to the tortured voice of a person in distress. I wondered to myself, as I had many times before, how many more stories like this one will I have to hear? When will hypoglycemia be accepted as a genuine and serious illness? My own experience and the experience of thousands of others demonstrate that hypoglycemia is real. It does exist. When will the medical profession take it seriously?

* * *

In 1980, when I formed the HSF, I wrote to about 50 local physicians looking for help and guidance. I was desperately seeking to arrange places to send the numerous patients who kept asking me where to go for treatment of their illness. No one responded. Discouraged and disillusioned, I decided to move beyond my local sphere of influence and contact physicians around the country who knew about hypoglycemia. Astonishingly, a number of them answered.

Emanuel Cheraskin, M.D., D.M.D., Harvey M. Ross, M.D., Jeffrey Bland, Ph.D., E. Marshall Goldberg, M.D., the late Carlton Fredericks, Ph.D. and the late Robert S. Mendelsohn, M.D., all responded, offering encouragement, support, guidance and hope. Although I was optimistic that I would hear from them, I think deep down inside I was surprised. Probably, because I knew the recent history of hypoglycemia. In the late 1960s and early 1970s, hypoglycemia was written up in a large number of lay publications. The disease suddenly became trendy. It was used as a way to explain some of the worst ills of humanity with little or no scientific backing, and a number of people proclaimed themselves to be hypoglycemics without bothering to consult a doctor or get a glucose tolerance test. The backlash in the medical establishment was swift. In 1949, the American Medical Association (AMA) awarded Dr. Seale Harris its highest honor for the research that led to the discovery of hypoglycemia. After the flood of quackery and self-diagnosis began, the AMA, in 1973, did a 180 degree turn and labeled hypoglycemia a "non-disease."

Don't let this discourage you. There are doctors out there. As the HSF started to gain recognition, acceptance and credibility, doctors from all fields of medicine volunteered their services. From general practitioners in the medical field to osteopaths, chiropractors, nutritionists, and dietitians, they all came. They lectured at our meetings, held seminars, wrote articles for our newsletters and served on our board of directors.

So, don't give up so easily. Take your time, have a positive attitude and follow the HSF's simple guidelines in your search for that special "healer."

Do ............. choose a physician carefully but preferably NOT during an emergency situation.

Do ............. ask for physician referrals from friends, neighbors, family, business associates, hospitals and organizations.

Do .............. read the chapter in this book on the glucose tolerance test, then call the office of someone you are considering and ask the following questions:

   a. Do you treat hypoglycemia?
   b. How do you test for it?
   c. If you administer the glucose tolerance test, how long does it take and how much does it cost?
   d. Do you provide nutritional counseling?
   e. What is your consultation fee?
   f. Are you available by phone if I need to reach you?
   g. Will you have time to answer any ques tions I may have?
   h. If I am having financial problems, will you take payments or will you accept my insurance? (ask only if applicable)

Do .............. have someone go with you on your first visit. Sometimes, the first visit is an emotional one and you may be nervous or apprehensive. Consequently, questions and/or answers may be misinterpreted or misunderstood. Having a second party along usually helps.

Do .............. bring a written list of symptoms, past medi-cal records and personal recollections relat-ing to your present problems. The impor-tance of your past history and the sequence of events leading up to your present condi-tion, cannot be overemphasized.

Do .............. bring in a diet/symptom diary (example in back of book). It should include a list of everything you have eaten, including any medication you may have taken in the previous five to seven days. Try to list the time eaten and any symptoms or reactions following consumption. This is important and can be a useful tool for the physician in diagnosing hypoglycemia. However, if you are physically and emotionally unable to do it, DO NOT PANIC -- a diagnosis can still be made without it.

Do .............. bring in your list of questions. Ask them one at a time and make sure you understand the answer before going on to the next.

Do .............. tell the physician about any medication you may be taking at the time. Certain medications cannot be tolerated by hypoglycemics.

Do .............. write down instructions of any kind, or take along a tape recorder.

Do .............. discuss in detail your feelings or concerns, not just your symptoms. If you have fears you are not expressing, your treatment will be longer, more difficult and far more expensive.

Do .............. be specific and to the point. The more prepared you are, the better equipped the doctor will be to make a proper diagnosis.

Do .............. find out if your physician is associated with a hospital in case of an emergency.

Do .............. discuss costs and insurance information.
Insurance companies differ on their policies
and willingness to pay for various tests and
procedures.  Is your doctor willing to work
out a payment arrangement and/or accept
whatever the insurance company pays?

Do .............. get a second opinion, especially if you are not
completely satisfied with the first physician.

Do .............. check the office procedures and staff.  Do
they overbook?  Are they friendly?  Are they
helpful?  The last thing you need is a doctor
too busy to listen or assistant who make you
feel uncomfortable.

Do .............. evaluate the doctor's office.  Is it clean and
neat?  Are the magazines up to date?  Is the
rest room adequately supplied?  An untidy
office and unstocked bathroom could mean
an indifference to cleanliness and to patients.
A nice assortment of current publications
may give you more confidence that the
doctor keeps him/herself informed and up to
date.

Do .............. take notice of the doctor's habits and appearance.  If the ashtray is full or if he/she is
severely overweight then their belief in (or
dedication to) good health practices should
be questioned.

Do .............. pay attention to your doctor's attitude,
attentiveness and professionalism.  Does he/

she give credence to your observations? Do they really take the time to listen?

Do ............... choose a competent, caring, and trustworthy physician who respects your individuality. The doctor-patient relationship is crucial. If your doctor doesn't have your complete confidence or isn't meeting your special needs, then it's definitely time to change.

Do ............... notify the physician's office, preferably in writing, if you are upset with the conduct or services of either the physician or the staff.

Do ............... discuss a complete prevention program. You need to know how to avoid future health problems, not just how to eliminate the ones you now have. Your current problems are not the only issues that need to be addressed.

Do ............... be leery of any alternative or new treatment that promises or claims to be a cure-all.

Do ............... wear a medic alert bracelet if you're experiencing many LBS symptoms; especially if you've recently blacked out or fainted. If your symptoms are under control you may keep your medic alert bracelet in your purse, car or briefcase - any place that can be seen in case of emergency. Medic Alert information is available at your local drug store or pharmacist.

\* \* \* \* \* \*

Don't .......... call your physician after listening or reading
an article on hypoglycemia and DEMAND a
glucose tolerance test. Instead, take this information, and a list of your symptoms and
the reasons why you feel the test is necessary.
Make an appointment to see your physician
and present him with all the information. If
he appears inattentive or cannot give you a
seemingly justifiable reason why you should
not have the test, look for another physician.

Don't .......... stay with a physician you cannot communicate with or feel confident about. It will only
complicate existing problems.

Don't .......... call your physician unnecessarily. If your
questions can wait, write them down and
save them for the next visit. The physician
will likely have more time then to give you a
better explanation.

Don't .......... wait to call your physician if you're in pain,
your symptoms are persistent, or last several
days.

Don't .......... continue to be a patient of any physician
who just listens for a few minutes and says
your symptoms "are all in your head." If you
are given a prescription for Valium, get a
second opinion as soon as possible.

Don't .......... withhold any medical history out of fear or
embarrassment. It is necessary for a proper
diagnosis.

Don't .......... seek the advice of a physician and then not follow the instructions issued to you. It's a waste of time and money.

Don't .......... run from one doctor to another. Give each one at least two to four visits to help you.

Don't .......... avoid going to a physician. If your symptoms persist after you've put yourself on a hypo-glycemic diet, seek medical advice.

Don't .......... avoid a physician because you lack insurance or money. Ask a family member or friend for financial assistance. You can't afford not to. If it is hypoglycemia, the faster you are diag-nosed and treated, the sooner you'll recover.

Don't .......... demand to be unnecessarily hospitalized.

Don't .......... hesitate to speak up - ask questions. If you're too timid or embarrassed to communicate with your doctor, then he/she won't be able to adequately meet your needs.

Don't .......... compare your program or progress with someone else's. Each person's emotional, physical and spiritual make up is unique. A competent physician will tailor a program to fit your individual needs.

Don't ......... forget, there ARE many caring, sensitive, trustworthy physicians out there. If at first you don't succeed in finding one - try, try again!!

# 5

## _The Importance of Individualizing Your Diet_

One of the HSF members called to tell me she was feeling terrible, particularly after eating breakfast. She started to shake, her stomach was nauseous and she felt jittery throughout the morning. She didn't understand why her symptoms were getting worse even though she was staying on a strict diet -- no sugar, white flour, caffeine, alcohol or tobacco.

I suggested that we go over her diet but she emphatically said, "It can't be my diet. I eat only what my doctor told me to eat and what the books I read suggested." However, upon my insistence, she started to give me an account of her daily intake of food. First thing every morning, she drank an 8-ounce glass of orange juice. Even though the book she read said to take four ounces, she figured eight should be twice as good.

I didn't let her continue any further. From my own personal experiences, there is no way I can handle orange juice on an empty stomach first thing in the morning. An 8-ounce glass of orange juice, although it is "natural," contains six teaspoons of sugar. For me and many hypoglycemics that I have spoken to, orange juice causes the same reaction as a strong cup of black coffee. The results are the shakes, butterflies in the stomach and an overall feeling of wanting to "jump out of your skin."

At first, it was difficult for this hypoglycemic to understand that if she had this "nervous attack" every morning after eating the same breakfast she should begin to question her diet; not continue to abide by it when she suffered adverse symptoms. We are individuals and thus must tailor every diet to our own bodies when a given diet proves troublesome.

As I mentioned before, there are many books on hypoglycemia. If you've read some of them, by now you're aware that many disagree on what type of diet to follow. It's indeed confusing if you read one book and it tells you to eat a high protein/low carbohydrate diet, while another book says to consume low protein/high carbohydrate foods. Where does that leave you, the confused and bewildered hypoglycemic?

First of all, I am sure that each author has enough confirmation and evidence that his or her diet is successful. Most likely, they all are. Probably, this is due to the fact that the big offenders (sugar, white flour, alcohol, caffeine and tobacco) are eliminated and six small meals are consumed instead.

But the key to a successful diet lies in its "individualization." Each one of us is different. Each one of us is biochemically unique. Therefore, every diet must be tailor-made to meet our individual nutritional requirements.

The list of foods your physician gives you or the list you may read in your favorite book on hypoglycemia, even the suggested food list in the back of this book, are basic guidelines. Variations come with time and patience, trial and error. Don't be afraid to listen to your body. It will send you signals when it cannot tolerate a food.

So, basically stick to the suggestions in the following do's and don'ts, and hopefully, with just a few adjustments during your course of treatment, a new and healthier you will gradually appear.

Do ............. keep a daily account of everything you eat for one week to ten days. In one column, list every bit of food, drink and medication that you take and at what time. In the second column, list your symptoms and the time at which you experience them. Very often you will see a correlation between what you have consumed and your symptoms. When you do, eliminate those foods or drinks that you notice are contributing to your behavior and note the difference. DO NOT STOP MEDICATION. If you believe that your medication may be contributing to your symptoms, contact your physician. A diet diary is your personal blueprint: a clear overall view of what you are eating, digesting and assimilating. It can be the first indicator that something is wrong and, perhaps, a very inexpensive way of correcting a very simple problem.

Do .............. start eliminating the "biggies" -- those foods, drinks and chemicals that cause the most problems: sugar, white flour, alcohol, caffeine and tobacco.

Do .............. be extremely careful when and how you eliminate the offending substances. Only YOU, with the guidance of a health care professional, can decide. Some patients choose to go at a steady pace. If you drink ten cups of coffee a day, gradually reduce consumption over a period of days or weeks. The same is true for food or tobacco. If you are heavily addicted to all of the aforementioned, particularly alcohol, then withdrawal should not be undertaken unless you are under the care of a physician.

Do .............. replace offending foods immediately with good, wholesome, nutritious food and snacks as close to their natural state as possible. Lean meats, poultry (without the skin), whole grains, vegetables and allowable fruits are recommended. We want to prevent deprivation from setting in, especially the "poor me, I have nothing to eat" attitude. There is plenty to eat.

Do .............. eat six small meals a day or three meals with snacks in between. Remember not to overeat.

Do .............. drink plenty of water. Most physicians say eight glasses of mineral water a day is best.

Do .............. be aware that when you start on a hypoglycemic diet, you might experience migrating aches, pain in your muscles and/or joints, headaches or extreme fatigue. This is normal when eliminating refined foods. Call your physician if they persist.

Do .............. be prepared to keep your blood sugar stabilized at all times, whether at home, office, school or traveling. At home you should always have allowable foods ready in the refrigerator or cupboards. Always keep snacks in your car or where you work.

Do .............. package food in Tupperware or air-tight containers. Aladdin's insulated thermos jar is handy for cold food and snacks. Aladdin also sells wide-mouth insulated bottles for hot foods, like soups or cut up meat and vegetables. Packaged nuts, seeds, rice cakes and cheese can be easily carried or stored in a purse or in jacket pockets. You can buy almost everything you need at a supermarket.

Do .............. rotate your foods. Eating the same foods over and over again for consecutive days can result in food sensitivities or allergies.

Do .............. read labels. Avoid ALL sugars -- dextrose, fructose, glucose, lactose, maltose and sucrose. Read labels in health food stores too. Just because you buy something in a health-food store, does not necessarily mean you can tolerate the ingredients.

Do .............. avoid artificial sweeteners, additives, preservatives and food coloring. Monosodium Glutomate (MSG) is a big problem for many hypoglycemics -- avoid it completely.

Do .............. watch your fruit consumption. If you are in the early or severe stage of hypoglycemia, you may not be able to eat any fruit. Some patients can eat just a small amount. Your diet diary will help guide you. Avoid dried fruits completely.

Do .............. be careful of the amount of "natural" foods or drinks you consume. Even though juices are natural, they contain high amounts of sugar. Whether or not the sugar you con-sume is natural, your body doesn't know the difference. Sugar is sugar is sugar and your body will react to an excess of it.

Do .............. dilute your juices, using about 2/3 juice to 1/3 water. If that's still too strong for you, try 1/2 juice and 1/2 water. Drink small quantities or drink them after you have eaten something, if you find that taking them on an empty stomach causes you problems.

Do .............. be inventive. Introduce new, unprocessed foods that have no preservatives, additives or chemicals. Look especially for grains and vegetables.

Do .............. arrange food to look palatable.

Do .............. broil, bake or steam food.

Do .............. attend some natural cooking classes. You will be taught to reduce sugar, salt, saturated fats, cholesterol and allergenic foods from your diet and still enjoy eating. Call your local schools, libraries and health food stores, or scan the local papers to find out what is available in your area.

Do .............. understand the meaning of "enriched." It does not mean extra amounts of vitamins. It means a small amount of some of the vitamins that were processed out of the food have been replaced.

Do .............. have your family stick to some of the basic principles of your diet. The big NO's for a hypoglycemic (sugar, white flour, alcohol, tobacco and caffeine) are detrimental to anyone's health.

Do .............. change your attitude about what constitutes a snack. We tend to think of snacks in terms of goodies or sweet treats. A good snack can be a half-baked potato with broccoli, half-stuffed tomato with tuna fish, some steamed zucchini and onions on a half cup of brown rice, a chicken leg or a slice of turkey.

Do .............. seriously consider going to OA (Overeaters Anonymous) or AA (Alcoholics Anonymous). Many HSF members found these meetings to be extremely helpful in controlling their addictions to sugar and food in general.

Do .............. be aware of the fact that some medications contain caffeine. If you're having reactions to the following medications, bring this matter to the attention of your physician: Anacin, APC, Caffergot, Coricidin, Excedrin Fiorinal, Four-Way Cold Tablets and Darvon Compound, etc.

Do .............. weigh yourself every day. Be aware of weight gain and weight loss. This is vital information in maintaining good health.

Do .............. check into other areas if you don't make progress with dietary changes. Hypoglycemia has been linked to allergies, hyperactivity, schizophrenia, juvenile delinquency, learning disabilities and candida albicans. Read the books recommended in the appendix for additional information.

Do .............. invest in the *Low Blood Sugar Cookbook*, by Edward & Patricia Krimmell. You can purchase it through Franklin Publishers by calling 215-525-1225.

Do .............. start a library of cookbooks. They don't necessarily have to be for hypoglycemics. Many good books with no or low sugar recipes are available.

Do .............. try at least one new recipe a week. At the end of the year you'll have tasted 52 new dishes, thus, ensuring that you are not tied to eating the same dull fare. It will help you look forward to mealtime and you won't feel so limited with your diet.

Do .............. store your food properly to avoid contamination and spoilage resulting from bacteria and molds.

Do .............. wash your fruits and vegetables thoroughly to reduce or remove the amount of pesticide residue.

Do .............. be aware that chemical sensitivities can aggravate LBS and induce reactions in vulnerable people. Paints, pesticides, solvents, gas stoves, smoke, even perfumes and hairsprays can make some people sick.

Do .............. know the seriousness of smoking cigarettes, especially for the hypoglycemic. According to our past Surgeon General, C. Everett Koop, "it is clear that nicotine in cigarettes and other forms of tobacco makes them addicting in the same sense as heroin and cocaine."

Do .............. also realize that alcohol is extremely dangerous to the hypoglycemic. If Alcoholism is an addiction you are experiencing, then you must read, *Under The Influence,* by Dr. James R. Milam and Katherine Ketcham.

*     *     *     *     *     *

Don't .......... panic when you first hear about all the foods that you must eliminate from your diet. Keep repeating all the foods that you CAN eat -- there are plenty.

Don't .......... stay on a diet that is not supervised by a professional, whether it's a physician, a nutritionist, or a holistic health practitioner. It should be someone with a degree or some training in nutrition.

Don't .......... forget that being PREPARED with meals and snacks is the key to a successful diet and a healthier you.

Don't .......... be apprehensive about eating out. Many restaurants now have salad bars, making it much easier for the hypoglycemic (just be sure to use either oil and vinegar or lemon juice for dressing). Lean meat, fish, vegetables and salad can be ordered at almost any restaurant.

Don't .......... skip breakfast. It's the most important meal of the day for a hypoglycemic.

Don't .......... worry unnecessarily about weight gain or loss at the beginning of the diet. As long as it is not severe and you are being supervised by a health care professional, it's common to have a weight fluctuation when the body is experiencing dietary changes.

Don't .......... compare your results or progress with anyone else's. Each body's metabolism is different.

Don't .......... take over-the-counter drugs or diet pills unless you have discussed this with your physician. They can have an adverse effect on hypoglycemics.

Don't .......... be obsessive about your diet. The CON-
STANT focus on what you can and cannot
eat will only instill more fear, stress and
frustration.

# 6

## _Glucose Tolerance Test_

So you think you may have hypoglycemia. You have all the symptoms. After discussing it with your physician, he agrees to give you a glucose tolerance test to confirm the diagnosis. A test for three or four hours is requested when diabetes is suspected, but a six-hour glucose tolerance test is by far the most reliable method to detect low blood sugar. You should settle for nothing less.

The night before having the GTT, you will be asked to fast after your evening meal. You are to eat or drink nothing until the time of the test. When you arrive at the doctor's office or laboratory, still fasting, a tube of blood will be drawn and you will be asked to give a urine specimen.

Then, you will be given a very sweet beverage called "Glucola" to drink. This drink contains a measured amount of glucose. Your blood will be drawn one-half hour later, and once again at one hour after drinking the Glucola. For each hour after that, you will give a blood sample until five or six hours have passed. A urine specimen is given each time your blood is drawn.

Each tube of blood and each urine specimen is tested to determine the amount of glucose it contains. When the report is sent to your doctor, he or she will be looking for glucose levels above or below normal at any time during the test.

During the test, you may start to sweat, get dizzy, weak or confused. If you experience these symptoms to the point of being extremely uncomfortable, or you get a headache or your heart starts beating quickly, ask the doctor's staff to draw your blood IMMEDIATELY. Any of those symptoms could be a sign that your blood sugar has dropped to a very low level, and you want you doctor to have the lowest readings possible. If you wait until the next hour, your blood sugar may go back up and your doctor will be deprived of information essential to making an accurate diagnosis.

The interpretation of the GTI is just as critical as its administration. Because individuals have different body chemistries, what is a normal drop or curve for one patient may not be for the next. Do not forget that laboratory tests are only aids to a diagnosis, not the final word.

Remember, too, that the test is not for everyone. Children and the elderly in particular frequently require another method. Dr. Carlton Fredericks, author of *Carlton Fredericks' New Low Blood Sugar and You*, frequently used "therapeutic diagnosis." "This means putting the suspected hypoglycemic on the correct diet and watching the response. If, after a month or two, the symptoms are significantly reduced, the diagnosis has been established." This procedure can be a less expensive, more convenient and less stressful method for diagnosing low blood sugar.

In conclusion, if you've read the basic facts about the glucose tolerance test, discussed it thoroughly with your physician and both of you have decided that this test is necessary, read the do's and don'ts first.

Do .............. understand the purpose, procedure and instructions BEFORE you have the glucose tolerance test administered.

Do .............. make sure the test is scheduled first thing in the morning (no later than 9:00 a.m.).

Do .............. ask the doctor or nurse to repeat instructions if you do not fully comprehend what you are or are not supposed to do.

Do .............. tell your physician, if he/she is not aware, if you are on any kind of medication. Some medications may affect blood sugar levels.

Do .............. use the "therapeutic diagnosis" for children and the elderly.

Do .............. bring someone with you, especially if you are experiencing severe symptoms.

Do .............. bring a book, newspaper or magazine of your choice to help overcome the boredom.

Sitting five or six hours is not something we're used to doing. Consequently, restlessness often sets in.

Do .............. have a pen and paper available to write down all the symptoms you are experiencing and at what time.

Do .............. bring a sweater with you. Very often, a patient will experience chills during the GTT. It is best to be prepared.

Do .............. arrange beforehand to have someone pick you up if you go alone for the test. Sometimes, afterward, you may be weak and driving could be difficult.

Do .............. bring a snack to eat immediately after the test, particularly if you must go home alone. Eating some protein (nuts, seeds, meat, cheese, etc.) will bring your blood sugar up, allowing you to feel good enough to get home safely.

Do .............. set up an appointment before you leave to go over your test results.

\*   \*   \*   \*   \*   \*

Don't .......... demand a glucose tolerance test. It is not always necessary.

Don't .......... accept a three or four hour glucose tolerance test for diagnosing hypoglycemia.

Don't .......... demand to have the glucose tolerance test if you have a fever or infection. It could affect the test results.

Don't .......... be shortchanged. Go over the results of your GTT with your physician thoroughly.

Don't .......... be fooled by the terms "borderline" or "mild" in the case of hypoglycemia. Too often when patients hear these terms, they don't take their diagnosis seriously. This could eventually cause grave consequences.

Don't .......... dismiss the fact that you may still be hypoglycemic even if the GTT doesn't confirm the diagnosis. Laboratory tests are not always conclusive. The conditions under which the test is given may alter the results. The best rule to follow is: don't treat the results of the test, treat the symptoms.

# _____Education A Must

L et's pretend it's your husband's birthday and you want
to surprise him with his favorite meal; veal cordon bleu.
It has been a while since you last made it. You have all the
ingredients but just don't remember how to make the stuff-
ing. Now you did have an excellent cookbook -- in fact,
that's where you got the instructions the first time. You'd
better find it.

Your anniversary arrives and you can't believe your
eyes. You're overwhelmed by the gift your family bought
you -- the food processor you always wanted. You just
can't wait for a special occasion or holiday so you can
show off your culinary skills. However, after you open up
the box and see all the pieces, you wonder, "Will I ever
learn to use them all? Does this food processor come with
a book? It must have directions."

It doesn't matter whether you're whipping up a gourmet meal, fixing a car, planting a vegetable garden or sitting down to learn how to operate a new computer, you need all the information and complete instructions BEFORE you begin.

You need to take the same kind of care with hypoglycemia. Read every book you can get your hands on that discusses the subject. Some will contradict each other, others will be confusing and difficult to understand. No matter. You will learn something from each of them. Remember, too, you don't have to read the thick books all at once, you can read them a chapter, a page or a few paragraphs at a time. Just do it consistently. Learning takes time, energy, patience and commitment. Don't give up. Just do it gradually and consistently. Don't say you don't have the time or ability; you do.

I wish I could personally introduce you to two HSF members who have taken "don't" out of their vocabulary. First there's Walter. Speak of determination! Here is a man who travels for more than 2 1/2 hours -- EACH WAY -- to attend our meetings. Walter is not sure how many miles he travels because he has to drive very slowly. Otherwise, his 1970 Ford pickup truck might not make it. When I asked him why he makes the trip every month, he didn't hesitate to respond, "Because I want to get better. I believe the meetings help me just like Weight Watchers helped my wife. Also, I have a lousy memory, so it's a reminder of what I have to do."

Then there's Hazel. I think she has attended almost every meeting the HSF has held in the last seven years.

I asked Hazel to share with you why she attended almost every meeting. "I was in terrible condition," she replied, "almost ready to commit suicide. In fact, at one point, I had a knife to my wrist. I threw it down and cried to my husband. . . he had to get me a doctor. I was confused, depressed, shaky. I was so angry because I couldn't do what I wanted to."

"I found a doctor in Beverly Hills. He took a glucose tolerance test but stopped it in the fourth hour because I was passing out. He was the first to tell me I was hypoglycemic but that I shouldn't worry. He recommended that I just eat candy, hard sour balls every hour, and go to see a psychiatrist. He also handed me the usual one-page diet. I locked myself in the house for a month. I didn't get off the couch. Then one day I read your article in "The Miami Herald." Since the diet the doctor gave me wasn't working and I was desperate, I attended the first HSF meeting."

I asked Hazel what the meetings had done for her. "They gave me the courage to stay on the diet," she said. "When I missed a meeting, I found that I would slip off my diet. I also learn something new every time I attend, even if it's only one thing. Sometimes I think I'm well and can do it alone, and then realize that I need support. You not only learn from each other, but you realize you're not alone."

It's not so important what method you use. Books, tapes, lectures -- they all give you the opportunity to learn, listen and share. Both Hazel and Walter can attest to this. I hope that one day you will, too.

Do .............. educate yourself about hypoglycemia. It is a
                  MUST in order to control your symptoms

and make the healing process as painless as possible. I cannot stress enough that KNOWLEDGE AND UNDERSTANDING OF THE CAUSES, EFFECTS AND TREATMENT OF THIS CONDITION ARE IMPERATIVE.

Do .............. start by getting a small library of books -- at least three -- by leading authorities in the field of hypoglycemia. (See the list of recommended books in the appendix). Then make it a habit to re-read them occasionally. You may find it more enlightening and informative on the second or third reading.

Do .............. remember to include in your library the LATEST books written on hypoglycemia. Diets change because of research in this field; therefore it is best to purchase some books that have been published in the last five years, or more recently. Use your public library or start a library with other hypoglycemics if cost is a factor. Sharing books will not only help monetarily but will open up doors of communication.

Do .............. buy yourself a marker and, while reading, mark any sentence that you feel applies to you and that you want to remember for fu-ture reference. Perhaps there is a sentence or paragraph that upsets or confuses you; mark it and discuss it with your physician or a health care professional working with hypoglycemic patients. Usually, just a simple explanation clears the way to a healthier you.

Do .............. realize that NO book will supply ALL the answers. Some, in fact, will be contradictory. Do take the information you feel you understand and apply it to yourself individually.

Do .............. consider tapes. For those who abhor the idea of reading, or who cannot read, for whatever reason, there are tapes available on hypoglycemia. These, fortunately, can be played anywhere at any time that's convenient.

Do .............. you suspect that your child, husband, wife, co-worker or friend is hypoglycemic? Are they reluctant to read any books or listen to tapes? If so, get some brief articles on the subject and leave them around the house, office or in their room. The bathroom mirror or the refrigerator door is an excellent place to start.

Do .............. attend meetings, lectures and seminars NOT ONLY on hypoglycemia, but on any health-related subject. Since most illnesses, such as heart disease, cancer, arthritis, diabetes, schizophrenia, are now being linked to improper diet, you are likely to get nutritional advice at any meeting you attend.

Do .............. your homework. Find out about such meetings through your local: newspaper, radio stations, TV (some early morning shows will list meetings), cable television, library, physician, health food store, hospital and Chamber of Commerce.

Do .............. contact your hospital, library or school. If no health-related meetings are scheduled, particularly on hypoglycemia, request that they consider the subject. This will alert your area to the needs and wants of the community.

Do .............. write down the date and time of the meeting, put it on your calendar, make arrangements with baby sitters, drivers and family members. Explain how important your attendance is at these meetings and prepare to swap services so that feelings of guilt or imposition do not arise.

Do .............. take your spouse or an immediate family member with you. It will take some of the pressure off the relationship if they understand the causes of your symptoms.

Do .............. use this time to share. If at first you're uncomfortable, try again at another meeting. Sharing experiences often relieves tension and fear, two emotions that can impede progress.

Do .............. have questions ready. Most meetings are followed by a question and answer period. Take advantage of this opportunity to gain invaluable information.

Do .............. be considerate if you have to use the restroom frequently or need to snack during the lecture.

Do .............. consider attending OA (Overeaters Anonymous) or AA (Alcoholics Anonymous). Even though they may not provide nutritional information per se, they will help you deal with addictive behavior. As hypoglycemics, we are addicted to certain foods -- white sugar and white flour are the biggest culprits.

Do .............. form your own support group, if nothing else is available. Two, three or four people gathered together, sharing and offering hope, can be the best medicine any doctor could prescribe.

*   *   *   *   *   *

Don't .......... pass up any opportunity to help make the journey back to health through information obtained at meetings, lectures and seminars.

Don't .......... give repeated excuses such as: I can't drive at night; it's too far; I can't get a baby sitter, etc. Perhaps the first time these excuses might be valid, but you should prepare for the next time.

Don't .......... ask questions that don't pertain to the subject during a meeting.

Don't .......... monopolize the floor. Give others a chance to speak.

Don't .......... surround the speaker before or after the program and try to get a diagnosis. Not only is it unfair to the speaker, but it can do you harm. It is impossible to make a diagnosis without a complete medical history and list of symptoms.

Don't .......... refuse to make a small donation if you are asked and can afford to. It is the only way that many of these meetings can continue.

# 8

_____*Are Vitamins Necessary?*

In 1984, I decided to leave my business partner, Marge, to give more time to the HSF. Our business was at the peak of its success. She and my husband were appalled that I would bow out, but I knew it was something I had to do.

When we were at the lawyer's office to sign the final papers, she seemed unusually upset. Her speech became slurred, she couldn't concentrate and she appeared lethargic. Her problems got worse and I became more alarmed. Although Marge was only in her mid-30s, she had suffered a stroke two years earlier, and I was worried that it might be happening again.

Questions poured out of me -- "Marge, why are you so nervous? Are you angry? Did you take a tranquilizer? Did you have a drink before you came here?" After throwing dozens of questions at her, I discovered the real culprit. Marge suffered from Premenstrual Syndrome (PMS) and was taking vitamin B-6 because she had heard that it could help control her symptoms. She bought a bottle of vitamins and, without knowing the proper dosage, began popping them into her mouth like gumdrops. She was overdosing on her vitamins.

In her effort to relieve pain, Marge, like so many of us, didn't bother to ask questions. She didn't take into consideration the proper dosage, the risk of allergic reactions, and the possible side-effects of combining medications with other vitamins or food. So desperate in her attempt to find a fast and easy cure, she did not even consider the potentially harmful consequences. Marge's poor judgment and inadequate information left her with an apprehensive and fearful decision about ever taking vitamins again.

This story is not unique. Situations similar to Marge's occur much too often. They breed controversy. Therefore, for every published article you read recommending the use of vitamins, be assured you will find a contrary view that discards them as nonessential.

The American Medical Association and the American Dietetic Association claim that if one consumes food from the four basic food groups and obtains the Recommended Daily Allowance (RDA), then the use of vitamins is unnecessary. But, who always eats a balanced diet?

Both associations feel that most Americans can and should get all the nutrients they need to be healthy from food rather than supplements. I don't think any advocate of supplements would disagree. However, what most Americans CAN and SHOULD do are not necessarily what they ARE doing. In fact, due to certain circumstances which I'll soon discuss, most Americans are nutritionally STARVED!! How? Read on.

Many of you have asked the question, "Do I need vitamins?" only to be told to just eat balanced meals. According to television commercials, one would tend to believe that a balanced meal consists of a hamburger, french fries and a coke.

Most of us are on a merry-go-round. Not the one for fun, but a merry-go-round of life; one that leaves us too busy and tired to get off and catch our breath. Many of us are faced with job and financial insecurities, family and marital difficulties, sickness, casualties and even death. It's no wonder that little time is spent on learning about the effects of poor dietary habits. Consequently, the diet of the 80s often consists of fast foods, heavily fried, sugar-laden, canned, frozen or leftover meals. Here lies just one of the many reasons why most people do not get sufficient amounts of vitamins and minerals in their diets.

Let's take into consideration some of the other vitamin "robbers:"

air pollution
alcohol
caffeine (coffee and soft drinks)
food additives, preservatives and food coloring
food processing
medication (Pill, diuretics, laxatives)
menstruation
soil depletion
stress (mental or physical)
tobacco

Examine the above list and review your dietary habits to see if you are eating a variety of fresh foods. Does your list include fresh vegetables, lean meats, whole grains and fiber?

What cooking methods do you use? Do you broil, steam or bake? How do you store your foods, particularly fruits and vegetables? All of these factors play a role in determining the amount of vitamins and minerals one actually consumes.

So, now, where does all this leave the hypoglycemic? Every book I've read on hypoglycemia and every doctor I've worked with over the past 13 years recommends vitamin and mineral supplementation for hypoglycemics. Vitamin therapy in conjunction with proper diet, exercise and reduction of stress has a positive, supportive and therapeutic effect in the treatment of hypoglycemia.

However, before you swallow that capsule, pill or liquid, read the following do's and don'ts:

Do .............. be informed and seek professional advice before starting any long-range, extensive vitamin therapy

Do .............. check out your local osteopathic physician, chiropractor, nutritionist or dietician if your present medical physician cannot supply you with this information. The aforementioned professionals are more likely to incorporate vitamin therapy as an adjunct to the healing process. Make sure the person you consult is licensed. Also try to speak to someone who has already used the practitioner's services and thus can give you insight as to their ethics, reputation and success.

Do .............. inform your physician if you are taking vitamins, especially if you are under that doctor's care for a particular disease or condition and/or are taking medication. Some vitamins and medications don't mix well and destroy or weaken each other's effects.

Do .............. check out the reputation of the vitamin store where you purchase your vitamins, especially if you're purchasing them without professional guidance. Ask questions about the vitamin or vitamins you are considering such as: What is the vitamin supposed to do? Should you expect side effects? How long should you take the vitamin? Is there any literature available on the product?

Do .............. make absolutely certain that the salesperson's first interest is in your health and safety and not in making a sale. If the salesperson has a forceful approach, leave and look for another store.

Do .............. check the price of vitamins. Once you know what you have to take, shop around for the best price.

Do .............. double check the dosage you are to take, the time of day it should be taken and any other instructions.

Do .............. check vitamin interaction. Avoid taking vitamins with alcohol or medication.

Do .............. make sure the vitamins you purchase haven't been tampered with. Check that the label hasn't been broken.

Do .............. .throw out any bottle whose label you are unable to read, either because it's faded or damaged.

Do .............. make sure the vitamins you purchase are not made with any fillers. There should be NO sugar, corn, wheat or starch.

Do .............. keep all vitamins in a cool place.

Do .............. keep vitamins out of reach of children.

Do .............. take vitamins with meals, unless otherwise directed.

Do .............. remember to take your vitamins with you on vacation and business trips. This is usually a time of increasing stress, strong activity and change of diet, and therefore not a good time to discontinue any program you are on.

Do .............. make it easy for yourself by carrying your vitamins in a carefree fashion. It is recommended that you try either a plastic container with compartments (you can purchase these at a drugstore or vitamin store) or zip-top plastic baggies. The latter are available in a size 2 X 2 inches. Old plastic prescription vials are also useful.

Do .............. STOP taking vitamins if you suspect them to be a cause of nausea, diarrhea, constipation, etc. You can introduce them at a later date, always one at a time. If there is still a reaction, STOP immediately.

Do .............. make sure you are absorbing your vitamins. Check your stool occasionally. If you can see a vitamin in its whole state, it is not being absorbed or assimilated in the intestinal tract. If that happens, talk to your physician.

\* \* \* \* \* \*

Don't .......... take vitamins indiscriminately! They can be just as harmful as medicine if taken without knowledge and caution.

Don't .......... double up on vitamins, thinking that if one is good, then two must be better. This is not necessarily so. Too many vitamins can be just as harmful as too much medication.

Don't .......... follow anyone else's vitamin program. You should have your own. REMEMBER: everyone is a unique individual with different needs. This individuality includes vitamin therapy of any kind, and therefore should be supervised by a professional.

Don't .......... run out and get the "vitamin of the month." Educate yourself before experimenting.

Don't .......... stop any medication abruptly because you start taking vitamins. Seek professional advice about combining the two.

Don't .......... stock up on vitamins. Your needs may change. Buy vitamins as you need them.

# _How Important Is Exercise?_

**H**ave you ever made a list of things you wanted to accomplish? I don't mean just a to-do list for next Monday, but a laundry list of goals that you want to achieve in your lifetime. I've written at least a dozen of these lists. At one point, I was adding one lifetime goal every day. I soon felt overwhelmed and frustrated because I knew I could not complete them all. I had to stop because I felt oppressed just thinking about the three dozen things I HAD to achieve in my lifetime.

No matter how ambitious my lists became, exercise was hardly ever on them, or if it was, it was near the bottom. This is probably because I was never athletic. I was born in Brooklyn, N.Y., in a six-family tenement house with no lawn or backyard. The nearest park was miles away. Skating was the only sports activity I participated in. There were plenty of schoolyards, sidewalks and empty streets around, but that was the extent of my exercise as a child. Some of my friends are still shocked when they hear I don't know how to ride a bicycle.

My attitude about exercise changed several years ago, when I attended a health seminar at which Covert Bailey, author of "Fit or Fat?" was one of the program speakers. After hearing him talk on the importance of exercise, I was totally convinced that I had to add exercise to my existing hypoglycemic regimen. I was controlling my hypoglycemia through diet and vitamins, but I knew I could fine-tune my physical condition, improve it, tone and strengthen my body if I incorporated specific daily physical activity into my life.

Now, you mention it and I've tried it; aerobics, yoga, stationary bike, mini-trampoline, jogging, swimming, jumping rope -- I've done them all. It was not until May 19, 1986, that I started walking. At first, I walked just a quarter of a mile, then a half mile and then, within a month, I was walking two miles a day, four to six days a week. This was a milestone for me. Walking has since given me more energy and flexibility, relaxes me better than any tranquilizer, suppresses my appetite and rejuvenates me both emotionally and physically.

Hopefully, it won't take you years of procrastination before you incorporate an exercise program into your daily life. Perhaps you can't do it now; you may be experiencing too many hypoglycemic symptoms. However, try making that list of goals as soon as you can. Just don't put exercise at the bottom.

The do's and don'ts of exercise are as follows:

Do ............... get your physician's approval before starting any exercise program. Most likely you will be given a complete physical, including an EKG and stress test, depending on your age, medical history and present symptoms.

Do ............... seek alternative advice from a health and fitness expert if you choose to ignore the above.

Do ............... choose your exercise carefully. The best exercises for hypoglycemics are: walking, swimming, dancing, jumping rope, riding a stationary bicycle and using a mini-trampoline. Walking is the most effective exercise, in addition to being the most compatible with normal daily activities. Depending on the stage of illness you are in, walking is the least stressful exercise for a hypoglycemic. Running, jogging or strenuous aerobic classes should be held off until most of the physical symptoms are controlled.

Do ............... seek a non-strenuous aerobic exercise program as an alternative to or in conjunction with walking.

Do ............... make sure the class you choose has an instructor who is qualified through both training and experience.

Do .............. check for information about time and date of classes, particularly free ones that are advertised in newspapers or community news bulletins.

Do .............. find a private instructor who will give you personalized lessons if you are afraid to start your exercise program with a group. Use the instructor until you are ready to join a group, which should be in a relatively short period of time. Yes, a personal instructor is expensive, but you will only be using that person for a short time. It is well worth the added expense.

Do .............. stretch before doing any exercise.

Do .............. switch exercises occasionally. It avoids over-development of certain muscles.

Do .............. a slower version of an exercise to warm up or cool down.

Do .............. be properly fitted with the appropriate clothing, depending on the exercise and climate. Avoid anything too heavy and tight in summer and too thin and flimsy in winter.

Do .............. be properly fitted with shoes.

Do .............. check the floor or exercise area for anything hazardous. For example, if you choose to skip rope, make sure the floor is not slippery or wet.

Do .............. consider a therapist who does body manipulation or deep muscle massage (osteopath, chiropractor or massage therapist) if sore muscles, malalignment of your body or torn ligaments prevent you from exercising. A massage therapist can produce better results than medication, a frequent foe of hypoglycemia.

Do .............. consider a "buddy system" if you need support or motivation to start a program. Grab your spouse or friend and begin together to reap the benefits of an alternative method to achieve good health and fitness.

Do .............. use every opportunity to increase your activity. Examples: Park in the far corner of the parking lot (during the day only) when shopping or going to work and walk those extra steps; pass up the elevator and take the stairs; and use a stationary bike or mini-trampoline while watching television.

Do .............. choose a role model to emulate. It needn't be a Jane Fonda, Rachel Welch or Jack LaLane. Sometimes a close friend will fit the bill. You should be comfortable with your choice.

Do .............. set aside a certain time or make a schedule for exercising. Its continuity on a regular basis, will assure success.

Do .............. make your exercise program FUN! Plan walking with a group of friends to a nearby mall or have a picnic near a lake or pool where later you can enjoy swimming, or, look into tennis lessons and bring along your favorite partner.

\*    \*    \*    \*    \*    \*

Don't .......... exercise just before bedtime. Exercise overstimulates the nervous system, making it difficult to unwind or relax.

Don't .......... choose an activity just because you think it'll burn the most calories. Selecting an exercise you don't enjoy will ensure defeat.

Don't .......... set high expectations. If you are leading a sedentary life, it would be unrealistic to walk one or two miles at first. You have to build up your stamina SLOWLY.

Don't .......... think you can lose weight quickly by pushing yourself to exercise too frequently. You'll only hinder any program you are on.

Don't .......... push yourself to exercise if you are too fatigued or are experiencing severe symptoms of hypoglycemia.

Don't .......... exercise on a full stomach.

Don't .......... exercise on a completely empty stomach, either. Eat an hour before exercising to avoid a blood sugar drop. Remember: don't eat a big meal; you should instead be eating several small meals throughout the day.

Don't .......... walk in hot sun, severe cold, or other undesirable conditions, such as rain, snow or strong winds.

Don't .......... wear tight clothes, especially zippers or buttons if you're in an exercise class where you must lie on your back or stomach.

Don't .......... .buy inexpensive shoes In the long run they'll cost you dearly .

Don't .......... compare your progress with someone else's. Each body is unique; therefore, length and success of each program is different.

Don't .......... give up too quickly on any program where you don't see results. Be PATIENT some programs don't result in a visible improvement for weeks or months.

# The Benefits
# Of Therapy

You found a doctor, took the glucose tolerance test and it's confirmed—you have reactive hypoglycemia. You begin to read about your condition, follow a diet, start on a vitamin program and, to your surprise, have enough energy to begin exercising. Even though your pace and timing may be slow at first, it's something you've never done before.

The severity of your symptoms starts to disappear. You're able to function—go to work, attend school and/or handle home situations. You should be thrilled. But you're not. You're full of fear, guilt and anger, and the loneliness is unbearable. You cry frequently. Discussing your feelings with family and friends only makes matters worse. Too often you hear remarks such as, "You should be grateful you only have hypoglycemia. Luckily, it's not cancer or a disease you could die from."

No, hypoglycemia will not kill you but, according to Dr. Harvey Ross, in his book, *Hypoglycemia, The Disease Your Doctor Won't Treat*, it's a disease that will make you wish you were dead.

Is there anything you can do? Yes. Maybe it's time to consider psychotherapy.

Although the attitude about seeking therapy is somewhat better, there are still many myths associated with this approach. At one time, it was considered only for people who were totally out of control, or for the severely mentally and emotionally ill. Consequently, people were afraid to open up, to share their inner most thoughts and secrets. If they did, perhaps some therapist would label them as "crazy," take control of their lives, put them away or do something else equally as bad.

Some people believe that nobody else ever has these feelings so therefore, no one else understands what they are going through. They fear exposing themselves and leaving themselves vulnerable.

Fortunately, for many, this thinking has changed. Today, it's not "Are you going for therapy?" but "Who are you going to?" Therapy, and there are many different types to choose from, has reached a level of acceptance. Some are seeking counseling to prevent minor problems from becoming major ones, some are seeking direction as to where they want to go in life, while others are trying to reclaim their lives entirely.

If you feel mentally and emotionally lost, if the physical problems of hypoglycemia are too much to bear, if you're ready to open up and discover the "real" you, and if you're ready to deal with all of those emotional issues in your life that you have put on the back burner, then thera- py may help you get back on the road to recovering from low blood sugar. Therapy does for the mind what diet and exercise do for the body. It's an investment that will pay dividends for the rest of your life.

Do .............. have a physical evaluation and any necessary tests to rule out a physical disease or condition before beginning extensive therapy.

Do .............. consider seeking therapy when the feeling of "I can't cope" arises. Waiting until an emergency or crisis, may force you into impulsive, short-sighted decisions.

Do .............. Look at therapy as a way to explore and discover yourself, especially if you are depressed and despondent.

Do .............. Look into the different types of therapy available from psychiatrists, psychotherapists, social workers, hypnotherapists and the clergy. Use the same criteria outlined in Chapter 3 on choosing a physician.

Do .............. be aware that therapists DO NOT have the answers to your problems. One of the things a therapist can do is to help patients to trust in their own thoughts and feelings, to explore them and to follow through in what they really WANT to do and not what they think they SHOULD do.

Do .............. search carefully for a competent therapist. Talk to friends. You'll be surprised to find

that many are seeking their advice and
guidance. Then, without prying into their
problems, ask questions: What do they like
or dislike about their therapist? Was he or
she helpful, and in what way? What benefi-
cial qualities did the therapists possess?

Do .............. evaluate the therapist, just as the therapist
evaluates you.

Do .............. find out:
1. where the therapist was trained,
2. the therapist's attitudes and points of view,
3. how the therapist plans to help you.

Do .............. see if you can develop a rapport with the
therapist. A trusting relationship between
patient and therapist is crucial to the healing
process.

Do .............. ask yourself, "Do I like this person? Am I
comfortable? Can I relate freely?

Do .............. be aware that finding a therapist is like
finding a marriage partner.  You have to
have faith, trust, open communication
and according to M. Scott Peck, M.D.,
author of *The Road Less Traveled*, "...the
essential ingredient of successful deep and
meaningful psychotherapy is love."

Do .............. realize that the spouse or significant other of
the hypoglycemic is under tremendous stress
and often needs therapy themselves. According to Dr. Hewitt Bruce, a psychologist in

West Palm Beach, Florida, that I have had the privilege of working with both personally and professionally, "No one understands the stress of the spouse or significant other. I believe that more than the patient, the spouse or significant other needs a lot of emotional support. They're not considered sick. They're not considered ill. They're healthy. They are strong. For the spouse it's sometimes a job to care for the hypoglycemic, yet there's no pay, no bonuses, no pat on the back and sometimes no appreciation. So many are suffering emotionally themselves and therapy of any kind could be of great value."

Do .............. consider group therapy. Many hospitals have programs to help patients deal more effectively with their emotions.

Do .............. remember that in any kind of group therapy confidentiality is crucial. It is the only way TRUST can be established, thus ensuring necessary success.

Do .............. check out the new holistic health centers for alternative methods if orthodox treatment fails to help. But be cautious of cultists or quacks.

Do .............. check your local papers for support groups that deal with mental or emotional problems.

Do .............. be fully aware of all the drastic effects of ECT (Electroconvulsive Shock Therapy), especially memory loss. If you're a computer expert, pharmacist, mathematician, etc., even a slight memory loss can deleteriously affect your life, endangering your livelihood.

Do .............. get a second opinion if ECT is prescribed or even suggested. Ask about other forms of treatment and give consideration to   there use. Remember— educating yourself about any treatment is crucial.

Do .............. realize that the end of therapy is, not only as important, but, sometimes more important than its beginning.

Do .............. read *"When To Say Goodbye To Your Therapist"*, by Catherine Johnson, Ph.D. It will help you determine whether you are treading water in therapy or whether you can strike out on your own.

\*    \*    \*    \*    \*    \*

Don't .......... look upon therapy as a sign of weakness. Remember, it takes more strength and courage to admit that you have problems and need help than to ignore the situation.

Don't .......... continue therapy if you feel you're not accomplishing something, even if only it's a small change or a little insight at each session.

Don't .......... blame yourself if:
      1. you feel extremely uncomfortable with the therapist,
      2. you feel intimidated,
      3. the therapist seems judgmental.

Don't .......... go back if the above feelings persist. Don't give up -- keep on looking.

Don't .......... stop therapy too suddenly. Give yourself sufficient time for treatment to become effective and gradually, as you grow more confident, wean yourself slowly from the therapist.

Don't .......... become so dependent on your therapist that you won't make a move without his/her direction.

Don't .......... panic if your therapist terminates the relationship. Sometimes, because of a sudden transfer, career change or ill health, your therapist must change his/her venue. Your present therapist should however assure you that he/she will put you in touch with another caring therapist.

# _Positive Attitude: It Won't Work Without It_

**W**hen I first began dreaming about forming the HSF, I was constantly plagued by my own insecurity. I wasn't a doctor, a nurse, or even a college graduate. What made me presume that I could start an organization to help sick people? I didn't have an answer to that question. Yet, there I was trying to form an advocacy group for a disease whose existence medical doctors didn't recognize, whose name most people couldn't pronounce and even fewer could understand.

What was worse, it wasn't even a disease with a lot of drama. It wasn't associated with children or death, and it wasn't even considered life-threatening. As a result, the media covered it only occasionally. How, I kept asking myself, can

I make people realize that low blood sugar is real, that the food/mood connection is real, that people can suffer severe emotional problems because their diet has thrown their body's chemistry out of balance?

I despaired of ever starting an organization which could have the kind of impact that would make people pay attention, especially because I didn't have any fancy titles or letters, such as Ph.D., after my name. Then, I started to read and re-read. My attitude started to brighten. I found out that many other lay people had contributed to the medical field. People such as Nathan Pritikin, founder of Pritikin Longevity Center; Jean Nidetch, founder of Weight Watchers; and Barbara Gorden, who wrote *I'm Dancing As Fast As I Can* and told the world about the dangers of Valium in a way no medical textbook ever could.

I knew there was hope. I began to visualize my dreams for the HSF. I wanted support groups in every state, a hypoglycemia hotline, visual aids in schools to warn children about junk foods, and proper testing for people being admitted to state mental hospitals, prisons, juvenile detention centers and jails.

What kept me going, and still does, is enthusiasm, positive thinking, positive people, faith, trust and a firm belief that this is a job that I have to do. It wasn't simple, not at first and not now. But it is getting easier, and it can get easier for you too. The tools, the people, the places, are all there to help. You just have to be ready to receive them. If you can't cope any longer with depression, guilt, fear and denial that a hypoglycemic confronts every day, then do something to replace these negative feelings with positive, uplifting ones.

Start by opening your hearts and minds to Dr. Wayne Dyer's books on positive thinking; Dr. Norman Vincent

Peale's on enthusiasm; Norman Cousins' on laughter; and Dr. Leo Buscaglia's on love. Mix them all together and let them be the cement that holds all the other necessary building blocks of good mental health together.

Do .............. have a support group of people who won't step on your dreams, who will encourage you, and support you emotionally when you're feeling good AND when you're not.

Do .............. have a good selection of positive reading material or tapes. Replacing bad feelings with positive ones is an arduous task. These tapes and books will help do the job when you need an ego boost and no one is around to give it to you.

Do .............. put up positive quotes around your house or office. They will lift your spirits and, as a bonus, they'll help lift the spirits of those around you.

Do .............. use positive words. Say "I can," "I will," and "I shall." Use only positive phrases, such as "This diet is working. It is the best I've ever had." Repeat these affirmations throughout the day.

Do .............. take 15 to 30 minutes every day for meditation or prayer. It refreshes the spirit.

Do .............. see happy, uplifting and funny movies. Laughter is terrific medicine.

Do .............. try yoga. It lowers blood pressure and relieves stress.

Do .............. consider listening to inspirational music, whether it's Bach or the Beatles.

Do .............. occasionally treat yourself to something special, whether it is lunch with a friend, a day on the golf course, a manicure, a massage, or a walk in the park.

Do .............. put your goals in writing. Read them over each day to instill a sense of purpose and direction. This way, you can check your progress and see that your goals are continuing to be met.

Do .............. stop procrastinating. If you've put off writing that letter, calling a friend, cleaning out your desk or closet or starting a project, do it NOW.

Do .............. seriously consider a job change if you've said more than once --- "I hate my job." Look into other fields than the one in which you are presently engaged. Learn what the requirements for employment are and take the necessary steps to get the training that's needed for this transition.

Do .............. seek intellectual stimulation. It enhances the body's immune function and helps increase your vitality. Try reading and/or attending

workshops and seminars on varied topics -
health, beauty, environment, business, etc.
Broaden your horizons and increase your
mental acuity.

Do .............. try to find a teenager, or use your own children, to do extra work around the house or
run errands.  Remember, you don't have to
be Super Mom or Dad!  You don't have to
do it all--or do it all alone.  Share the load of
responsibilities.  You'll be surprised at how
well someone else can do these tasks!

Do .............. volunteer work. Many times in helping
others, we end up helping ourselves.

*     *     *     *     *     *

Don't .......... surround yourself with people who have
nothing but negative things to say about the
world and what you are trying to achieve.
They'll only make reaching your goals more
difficult.

Don't .......... use the words "can't" and "won't " Negative
words produce negative thinking.

Don't .......... watch depressing movies or listen to sad
music when you feel depressed It will only
make you feel worse.

Don't .......... see problems as obstacles. See them as a way
to learn and grow.

Don't .......... worry so much about the future or dwell on
the past that you miss out on "living" today.

# _Health and Beauty: You Can't Have One Without The Other

I'd like to mention a special someone who, because of her faith and trust in my work and reputation, chose me to assist her in a once-in-a-lifetime assignment. Carolyn Stein, president of Carolyn Stein & Associates, is a media image consultant. She is called upon to create an image of success and to develop top communication skills through her workshops, seminars and keynote speaking engagements.

Every four years, for the past sixteen years, Carolyn has been given a very special assignment...media image consultant to the Republican National Convention. This year, I went as her assistant.

Carolyn was aware of my previous work in the beauty industry and knew that I now devoted most of my time and energy to the HSF and the Florida Speaker's Association, of which she and I were both directors. It didn't take much persuasion, though, for Carolyn to convince me to go along as her assistant on what was indeed going to be the ultimate "special assignment".

We arrived in Houston, Texas, on August 14th. By the time I left one week later, I would have shaken hands and rubbed elbows with three Presidents of the United States and their First Ladies, the present Vice President and his wife, the President's Cabinet and Senators and Representatives from all over the country. Add to that list stars like Tanya Tucker, Wynonna Judd, Gerald McRaney, the Gatlin Brothers, Roger Staubach and Lee Greenwood.

There I was, Roberta Ruggiero. Whether I was applying make-up, re-doing a hairstyle or straightening out a jacket or tie, I was taking part in American history! It was phenomenal!

However, I kept asking myself, "Why me?...Why had I been chosen for this special assignment?" Particularly, since most of my work is in the health field. Well, ask a question, and if you stop long enough to listen, there's always an answer.

I have repeatedly said health and beauty go hand and hand. You can't have one without the other. So, there I was, right smack in the middle of proving my theory correct. Everyone with whom I came in contact had a "glow".

I saw skin, hair and nails ...the picture of health. I felt energy, vitality and excitement emanating from all those in the vicinity. It was clearly evident that the health and beauty, honor and pride of each individual present would be a contributing factor to the success of this convention.

The experience in Houston confirms what I have been saying all along...diet ALONE does not control low blood sugar symptoms. Besides individualizing your diet to your particular needs, you must look into a vitamin program, an exercise regimen and stress reduction techniques. You need to maintain a positive attitude, associate with positive people and look to meditation and prayer for an inner source of peace and fulfillment. And last, but not at all least, you must take a look at your physical beauty. It's all there, ready to shine. Enhance it a bit with a new hairstyle; give yourself a facial or a manicure and pedicure. Be daring; spruce up some old outfits with scarves, pins, fashion earrings or belts. Buy that wild tie you've always wanted or the boots you felt too embarrassed to wear.

Health and beauty...it's so important to look it, feel it and be it. Combine the two...you never know where it could take you. It took me to Houston!

Do .............. remember this chapter is to spur you on; to start the wheels going and your enthusiasm flowing. It is just a prerequisite for you to look further into whatever area sparksyour interest.

Do .............. set a special "beauty" time aside each week just for you. A time to focus and enjoy the art of taking care of your personal needs. A time to pamper yourself from head to toe. You've been worried about what you put INSIDE your body; it's now time to take care of your outward appearance.

Do .............. buy some books or magazines on beauty.
They will give you more in depth explanations of the areas I've highlighted in the
following do's and don'ts. If money is a
problem— spend some time at your local
library—they usually have the most up-to-
date beauty publications.

Do .............. start your beauty session with a long, relaxing
bath. Light some candles, burn some incense
and put on some soft music. Let this be some
private time just for you.

Do .............. try some aromatherapy in the bath. According to aromatherapist, Gerri Whidden,
"Aromatherapy is the use of natural plant
essence to produce health, beauty and well
being. A few drops of the essences called
Essential Oils can  be used for inhalation in a
bath or as massage oil to stimulate, sedate or
uplift."

Do .............. try a loofah scrub brush, and use it after
soaking in the bath. Wet the loofah with
soap and, using a circular motion, massage
your skin.  It'll remove dry, dead cells and
make your skin feel soft as silk. The loofah
scrubs are inexpensive and can be purchased
at your local beauty supply or drug store.

Do .............. give yourself a manicure after a bath or
shower. Your cuticles will be soft and easier
to push back. First, file your nails GENTLY

with an emery board. Take your time to acquire the shape you desire. Make sure that you don't file too much into the nail corners. This weakens the nail.

Do .............. push back your cuticles GENTLY and do not use a nail file. Use an orange wood stick. It is even better to cushion the end of the stick with a little cotton. This will allow you to put pressure on the cuticle yet not cause any pain or injury.

Do .............. invest in a pumice stone especially designed for the tip of the nail. This will smooth the nail and give you a better looking manicure. Again, this is inexpensive and can be purchased at your local beauty supply store or drug store.

Do .............. trim excess cuticles and hangnails CAREFULLY with a cuticle nipper.

Do .............. massage your hands with cream. Wipe off the cream that is on the nails. This can be done by using a cotton ended orange wood stick which has been dipped in polish remover. Go over the nail gently, and remove any excess cream or polish.

Do .............. apply a base coat. This is absolutely necessary for the nail polish to adhere to the nail. Otherwise, your polish will start to wear off immediately. Then apply two thin coats of your desired color of polish. WAIT as long as you can before applying a top coat. If all these coats of polish are put on without allowing them time to dry between coats, your polish will NEVER fully set.

Do .............. apply a soft new shade or try a wild romantic color to your nails, even if you've never done it before. I promise it'll perk you up!

Do .............. give yourself a pedicure using the same steps as above.

Do .............. treat yourself to a professional manicure and pedicure. Your birthday or anniversary is the perfect time to indulge yourself.

Do .............. treat yourself to a professional facial by a licensed aesthetician at least once or twice a year. In between, a minimum of once a month, give yourself a home facial.

Do .............. start by choosing the best facial products for you. It's very hard to recommend a product but, again, a licensed aesthetician would be able to help you decide what's best for your skin type and tone. If an aesthetician is not available in your area, go to a cosmetic counter at your nearest department store.

Do ............. start with a cleanser that will remove all residue as the first step of your facial.

Do ............. follow it with a deep pore cleanser. Remember to be very gentle with your skin. Don't pull or push it.

Do ............. use a gentle mask specially chosen for your skin type. Rinse thoroughly. The rinsing process is extremely important. Gently pat dry and use a protective day or night cream.

Do ............. remember that consistency is of the utmost importance. Continually starting and stopping any program on health or beauty is most deleterious to your body. It sends mixed signals and can cause undue stress.

Do ............. seriously consider a make-up session with a professional cosmetologist. It will enhance your appearance and do wonders for your morale.

Do ............. be aware that according to research, cosmetic allergies can also lead to hay fever and asthma. Discuss this with your physician if you feel this may apply to you.

Do ............. consider a hair removal process, either waxing or electrolysis, if excess facial or bikini hair a source of discomfort or embarrassment. Consult a licensed aesthetician in your area for a professional evaluation.

Do .............. consider a professional massage.  Massage Therapist, Judith McBride, R.N., L.M.T., says, "It is my experience that massage therapy is an excellent way to help nurture and heal others. I have found that by restoring balance through the physical being, the mental, emotional and spiritual self are positively influenced. As a Nurse Massage Therapist, I have effectively blended several disciplines to serve as a natural method for wellness by facilitating healthier lifestyle choices and illness/injury prevention."

Do .............. be aware that the benefits of Massage Therapy include: deep relaxation and stress reduction, relief in muscle tension and stiffness, increase in circulation of both blood and lymph fluids and an over-all increase in flexibility and coordination.

Do .............. consider a new hairstyle—sometimes a new look is a great image booster and morale energizer.  However, remind your hairstylist that you want a hairstyle that is simple, uncomplicated and requires light maintenance.

Do .............. talk to your hairstylist about a permanent. This can add fullness, body and manageability to fly-away, baby-fine or coarse hair.

Do .............. consider cosmetic dentistry -- bonding or veneer covering if the appearance of your

teeth is causing you shame and embarrassment - or even if you just want to improve
your appearance. Seek out professional
advice from your local dentist.

Do .............. buy a new item for your wardrobe— a shirt, a
blouse, a new tie. Be daring—buy and wear
what you've always wanted to wear but
were too afraid or ashamed to try. Do it—do
it now!

Do .............. put sleep high on your priority list. It's
extremely imperative to get a sufficient
amount of sleep. It is during the sleep period
that the healing process is accelerated.

Do .............. try stress reducing techniques when falling
asleep is difficult—deep breathing, medita-
tion, yoga, stretching, or a hot bath. Put
on soft music, read a book — whatever
kind relaxes your mind, have sex — only
if consensual.

*   *   *   *   *   *

Don't .......... sit in the sun and bake because you think a
tan will make you look healthy. You'll pay a
price—dry, wrinkled skin, plus an increased
risk of developing skin cancer.

Don't .......... pull, push, poke or squeeze your skin at any time, especially if you have a blemish on your face. You could cause permanent scarring or accelerate the stretching and aging of the outer layer of your skin.

Don't .......... wear tight clothing, especially belts, shoes or pants. Avoid any unnecessary discomfort.

Don't .......... underdress in winter or cold weather or overdress on hot summer days. Again we want to avoid severe changes in body temperature.

Don't .......... continue using any make-up or skin care product if you experience any allergic reactions. Consult an aesthetician or dermatologist for advice and direction.

Don't .......... take too hot a bath or soak too long. It could leave you weak. If you're experiencing many hypoglycemia symptoms it is best not to take a bath unless someone else is at home with you in case an emergency arises.

Don't .......... use a sauna, hot tub or jacuzzi unless you use precaution. Please follow posted instructions. If you are experiencing a host of symptoms do NOT use prior to consulting your physician.

**Don't** .......... have hair removal done - whether waxing, electrolysis or even tweezing—during your menstrual cycle. The outer layer of the skin is very sensitive during this time and often contributes to more pain and sensitivity than usual. If you must tweeze eyebrows—try applying some baby Oragel first—it'll slightly numb the skin and help to lessen the pain. This is an excellent tip for teenagers having their eyebrows done for the first time.

**Don't** .......... attempt a manicure or pedicure if you have difficult or fungus nails. See a licensed manicurist or pedicurist or licensed podiatrist.

**Don't** .......... .think for a moment that all of the above do's and don'ts apply only or mostly to women. Today, many men are removing the barrier of "for women only" and enjoying and benefitting from the combination of health and beauty techniques. Be brave men— give some of this a try!

# _Hypoglycemia Questionnaire/ Symptom Diary_

## Hypoglycemia: Do You Have It?

In the space provided below, please mark ( 1 ) if you have this condition mildly, (2) if moderate, and (3) if severe. If you do not have the condition, leave it blank. The accuracy of this questionnaire depends upon complete honesty and serious objective thought in answering the questions. (Many of these symptoms may relate to other health problems).

1____Abnormal craving for sweets
2____Afternoon headaches
3____Allergies: tendency to asthma, hay fever, skin rash, etc.
4____Awaken after a few hours sleep/difficulty getting back to sleep

5____ Aware of breathing heavily
6____ Bad dreams
7____ Blurred vision
8____ Brown spots or bronzing of skin
9____ "Butterfly stomach," cramps
10____ Can't make decisions easily
11____ Can't start in morning before coffee
12____ Can't work under pressure
13____ Chronic fatigue
14____ Chronic nervous exhaustion
15____ Convulsions
16____ Crave candy or coffee in afternoons
17____ Cry easily for no apparent reason
18____ Depressed
19____ Dizziness, giddiness or light-headedness
20____ Drink more than 3 cups of coffee or cola a day
21____ Get hungry or feel faint unless eat frequently
22____ Eat when nervous
23____ Feel faint if meal is delayed
24____ Fatigue relieved by eating
25____ Fearful
26____ Get "shaky" if hungry
27____ Hallucinations
28____ Hand tremor (or trembles)
29____ Heart palpitates (beats fast) if meals missed or delayed
30____ Highly emotional
31____ Nibble between meals because of hunger
32____ Insomnia
33____ Inward trembling, feels better after meals
34____ Irritable before meals
35____ Lack of energy
36____ Moods of depression, "blues" or melancholy
37____ Poor memory or ability to concentrate
38____ Reduced initiative

39____Sleepy after meals
40____Sleepy during the day
41____Weakness, dizziness
42____Worrier, feel insecure
43____Symptoms come before breakfast
44____Total Score.

Add the total of all answers. A total score of less than (20) twenty is within normal limits. A higher score is evidence of probable adrenal insufflciency and/or deranged carbohydrate metabolism (Hypoglycemia), and would indicate further testing.

# DIET-SYMPTOMS-FEELINGS DIARY

Record your menus, snacks, medications and the time
you take them along with any significant feelings and symptoms in one or two word statements.

| TIME | FOOD-DRINK-MEDICATIONS | TIME | SYMPTOMS & FEELINGS |
|------|------------------------|------|---------------------|
|      |                        |      |                     |
|      |                        |      |                     |
|      |                        |      |                     |
|      |                        |      |                     |
|      |                        |      |                     |
|      |                        |      |                     |
|      |                        |      |                     |
|      |                        |      |                     |
|      |                        |      |                     |
|      |                        |      |                     |
|      |                        |      |                     |
|      |                        |      |                     |
|      |                        |      |                     |
|      |                        |      |                     |
|      |                        |      |                     |
|      |                        |      |                     |
|      |                        |      |                     |
|      |                        |      |                     |
|      |                        |      |                     |
|      |                        |      |                     |
|      |                        |      |                     |
|      |                        |      |                     |
|      |                        |      |                     |
|      |                        |      |                     |
|      |                        |      |                     |
|      |                        |      |                     |
|      |                        |      |                     |
|      |                        |      |                     |
|      |                        |      |                     |
|      |                        |      |                     |

*Recommended Foods/Menus*

## RECOMMENDED FOODS

*Note: The following list of recommended foods and menus is just a guideline. You must remember that everyone's body chemistry is different, therefore, adjustments must be made to meet individual need. Size of portions depend on weight and symptoms. READ the chapter on INDIVIDUALIZING YOUR DIET before incorporating the menus into your diet program.*

Meats:      All kinds of fresh meats—veal, lamb, lean beef, pork (if no nitrates).

Poultry:    Without skin—chicken, turkey, Cornish hens, duck, pheasant.

| | |
|---|---|
| Fish: | Flounder, turbot, sole halibut, grouper, cod, hadock, salmon, red snapper, scallops, tuna, shrimp, lobster, crab. |
| Dairy | Whole milk, skim milk, cheeses (farmer, cot tage, ricotta, mozzarella), eggs, butter and yogurt. |
| Grains: | 100 percent whole wheat bread, brown rice, millet, oatmeal, buckwheat, oats, whole wheat pasta and noodles. |
| Nuts and Seeds: | Almonds, cashews, walnuts, pecans, chestnuts, sunflower seeds, pumpkin seeds. |
| Vegetables: | Artichokes, asparagus, avocado, beans, beets, broccoli, brussel sprouts, cabbage, carrots, caulillower, celery, chives, collard, corn, cucumber, eggplant, endive, garlic, kale, lettuce, mushrooms, mustard greens, okra, onion, parsley, peas, peppers, potatoes, pumpkin, radish, rhubarb, spinach, sprouts, tomatoes, zucchini, yams. |
| Beverages: | Water, vegetable juice, herbal tea, seltzer, clear broth. Occasionally, decaffeinated coffee or weak tea. |
| Fruits: | Avocado, strawberries, apples, peaches, pears, oranges, watermelon, tangerines, berries, plums, grapefruit, honeydew. |

# FOODS TO AVOID

Desserts:
Anything containing white sugar, such as, candy, cakes, pastries, custard, Jell-o, ice cream, sherbet, pudding, cookies, breakfast cereals, and commercially baked breads. Avoid honey and other forms of sugar, such as brown, raw, and turbinado.

Grains:
Anything containing white flour, such as packaged breakfast cereals, gravies, white rice, refined corn meal, white spaghetti, macaroni, noodles and refined bakery goods.

Meats:
Lunch meats, bacon, sausage, processed meats (most contain corn sugar), meat or meat products with artificial colors, flavorings or preservatives.

Beverages:
Alcohol and caffeine and all sugared soft drinks and fruit juices.

Fruits:
Dried fruits (figs, dates, raisins). Fruit juices can be tolerated at times if diluted. Avoid EXCESSIVE amounts of fresh fruit.

*Note: Tobacco should be avoided entirely.*

# SUGGESTED LIST OF SNACKS

FRESH VEGETABLES: tomato wedges, sliced cucumbers, carrot and celey sticks, radish flowers, sliced summer squash, and zucchini, cauliflower and broccoli flowerettes (steamed) mushrooms, pepper rings.

FRESH FRUIT: apple wedges orange slices, cantaloupe, watermelon, strawberries (in moderation)

COTTAGE CHEESE
HARD BOILED EGG
YOGURT
GRANOLA SEEDS (sesame, sunflower, pumpkin)
NUTS (almonds, cashews, pecans, walnuts)
POPCORN
COLD CHICKEN, TURKEY, ROAST BEEF
CHEESE SLICES
WHOLE GRAIN BREAD (with nut butter)
RICE CRACKERS (with natural peanut butter, tuna fish or
    cheese)
RICE WAFERS (with natural peanut butter, tuna fish or
    cheese)
WHOLE WHEAT PRETZELS
APPLESAUCE (no sugar)
CELERY STICKS (stuffed with peanut butter, tuna fish or
    cheese)
BAKED POTATO (with steamed vegetables)

# SUGGESTED BREAKFASTS

1/2 cup of oatmeal
1 poached egg
1/2 grapefruit
Beverage

1 egg omelet with green peppers, onions or mushrooms
1 slice whole wheat bread or rice cake
1 orange
Beverage

1/2 cup of cream of rice (millet, grits, dry rolled oats)
· Cheese omelet
1 cup strawberries
Beverage

1 - 2 slices of whole grain bread
1 cup cottage cheese
Beverage

# SUGGESTED LUNCHES
# AND DINNERS

Chef salad (egg, turkey, chicken, lettuce, carrots, etc.), with oil
      and vinegar dressing
1 slice whole wheat bread or rice cake
Beverage

Soup (bean, lentil, chicken or beef
Small tossed salad
1 slice whole wheat bread
Beverage

4 - 6 oz. broiled shrimp (or fish of any kind)
Green beans with almonds (or mushrooms)
Small tossed salad
Beverage

4 - 6 oz. chicken (one leg, thigh or breast)
1 small potato
Broccoli
Small tossed salad
Beverage

Broiled lamb chop
Brown rice
Brussel sprouts
Small tossed salad
Beverage

# A FINAL NOTE

This book is just meant to be the beginning. It was written with the hope of sparking your enthusiasm, planting the seed of hope and giving you the strength to continue learning, seeking and finding the answers to controlling low blood sugar.

Continue gaining knowledge. This, in turn, will give you the wisdom and courage to grow in every area of your life— physically, mentally, emotionally and spiritually. It is only by healing the "total" body that you can achieve optimum health.

# APPENDIX A

## ———— *Recommended Books On Hypoglycemia*

*Body, Mind and Sugar,* by E.M. Abrahamson, M.D. and A.W. Pezet. New York, Avon Books, 1977.

*Carlton Fredericks' New Low Blood Sugar and You,* by Dr. Carlton Fredericks. NewYork, Perigee Books, 1985.

*Food, Mind and Mood,* by David Sheinkin, M.D., Michael Schacter, M.D., and Richard Hutton. New York, Warner Books, Inc., 1979.

*Fighting Depression,* by Harvey Ross, M.D., New York, Larchmont Books, 1975.

*The Hidden Menace of Low Blood Sugar,* by Clement G. Martin. New York, Arco Publishing Co., 1976.

*Hypoglycemia: A Better Approach*, by Paavo Airola, Ph.D.
Phoenix, Health Plus Publishers, 1977.

*Is Low Blood Sugar Making You a Nutritional Cripple?* by
Ruth Adams and Frank Murray. New York, Larchmont
Press, 1970.

*Lick The Sugar Habit*, by Nancy Appleton, Ph.D. New
York, Warner Books, Inc., 1986.

*Low Blood Sugar Handbook*, by Ed and Patricia Krimmel. Bryn
Mawr, PA, Franklin Publishers, 1984.

*Low Blood Sugar; What it Is and How to Cure It*, by Peter J.
Steincrohn, M.D., Chicago, Ill., Contemporar Books,
Inc.,1972.

*Nutraerobics*, by Dr. Jeffrey Bland, New York, Harper and
Row, 1983.

*Psychodietetics*, by Emanuel Cheraskin, M.D., D.M.D.,
William Ringsdorf, Jr., D.M.D. with Arline Brecher. New
York, Bantam    Books, 1978.

*Sugar and Your Health*, by Ray C. Wunderlich, Jr., M.D. St.
Petersburg, FL, Good Health Publications, Johnny Reed,
Inc., 1982.

*Sugar Blues*, by William Dufty. New York, Warner Books,
Inc., 1975.

*Sugar Isn't Always Sweet*, by Maura (Jinny) Zack and
Wilbur  D. Currier, M.D. Brea, CA, Uplift Books, 1983.

*Sweet and Dangerous*, byJohn Yudkin, M.D. New York,
Bantam  Books, 1972.

# COOKBOOKS FOR THE HYPOGLYCEMIC

*The Allergy Cookbook,* by Ruth R. Shattuck. NewYork, A Plume Book, 1984.

*Cooking Naturally For Pleasure and Health,* by Gail C. Watson. Davie, FL, Falkynor Books, 1983.

*Foods For Healthy Kids,* by Dr. Lendon Smith. New York, Berkley Books, 1981.

*Hypoglycemia Control Cookery,* by Dorothy Revell. New York, Berkley Books, 1973.

*The Low Blood Sugar Cookbook,* by Francyne Davis. New York, Bantam Books, 1985.

*Dr. Lendon Smith's Diet Plan For Teenagers,* by Lendon Smith, M.D. NewYork, McGraw-Hill, 1986.

*Step-By-Step To Natural Food,* by Diane Campbell. Clearwater, FL, CC Publishers, 1979.

*Sugar Free. . .That's Me,* by Judith S. Majors. New York, Ballantine Books, 1978.

*The Low Blood Sugar Cookbook,* by Ed and Patricia Krimmel, Bryn Mawr, PA, Franklin Publishers, 1984.

# EXERCISE BOOKS FOR THE HYPOGLYCEMIC

*Aerobics,* by Kenneth H. Cooper, M.D., NewYork, Bantam, 1972.

*Aerobics For Women*, by Kenneth H. Cooper, M.D., New York, Bantam Books, 1973.

*The Aerobics Program For Total Well-Being*, by Kenneth H. Cooper, M.D., New York, Bantam, 1983.

*The Complete Book of Exercisewalking*, by Gary D. Yanker. Contemporary Books, Inc., 1983.

*Fit or Fat?* by Covert Bailey. Boston, Houghton Mifflin Company, 1977.

Gary Yanker's *Sportwalking*, by Gary Yanker, New York Contemporary Books, 1987.

# BOOKS TO HELP DEVELOP
# A POSITIVE ATTITUDE

*Anatomy of An Illness*, by Norman Cousins, New York, W.W. Norton & Co., 1979.

*Bus 9 To Paradise*, by Leo Buscaglia, New York, Fawcett, 1987.

*Enthusiasm Makes the Difference*, by Norman Vincent Peale, NewYork, Fawcett, 1987.

*Gifts Form Eykis*, by Dr. Wayne Dyer, New York, Pocket Books, 1983.

*Goodbye to Guilt*, by Gerald G. Jampolsky, M.D., New York, Bantam Books, Inc., 1985.

*The Healing Heart*, by Norman Cousins, New York, Avon Books, 1983.

*Love,* by Leo Buscaglia, New York, Fawcett Crest Books, 1972.

*Loving Each Other,* by Leo Buscaglia, NewYork, Fawcett Columbine, 1984.

*Personhood,* by Leo Buscaglia, New York, Fawcett Columbine, 1978.

*The Power of Positive Thinking,* by Norman Vincent Peale, NewYork, Prentice-Hall, Inc., 1952.

*Pulling Your Own Strings,* by Dr. Wayne Dyer, New York, Thomas Y. Crowell Co., 1978.

*The Road Less Traveled,* by M. Scott Peck, M.D., New York, Simon and Schuster, 1978. ]

*Tough Times Never Last, But Tough People Do!,* by Robert H. Schuller, NewYork, Bantam Books, 1983.

*The Sky's The Limit,* by Dr. Wayne Dyer, New York, Simon and Schuster, 1980.

*Teach Only Love: The Seven Principles of Attitudinal Healing,* by Gerald G. Jampolsky, M.D., New York, Bantam, 1983.


*When Bad Things Happen to Good People,* by Harold S. Kushner, New York, Avon Books, 1981.

*Your Erroneous Zones,* by Dr. Wayne Dyer, New York, Funk & Wagnalls, 1976.

# BOOKS ON THE CORRELATION BETWEEN HYPOGLYCEMIA AND LEARNING DISABILITIES, JUVENILE DELINQUENCY, MENTAL ILLNESS, ALCOHOLISM AND CANDIDA ALBICANS

*Allergies and the Hyperactive Child*, by Doris J. Rapp, M.D. NewYork, Simon & Schuster, 1979.

*Brain Allergies*, by William H. Philpott, M.D. and Dwight K. Kalita, Ph.D. New Canaan, CT, 1980.

*Chocolate to Morphine*, by Andrew Weil, M.D., and Winifred Rosen. Boston, Houghton Mifflin, 1968.

*Diet, Crime and Delinquency*, by Alexander Schauss, Berkely, CA, Parker House, 1981.

*Eating Right To Live Sober*, by L. Ann Mueller, M.D., and Katherine Ketchum, NewYork, NAL, 1986.

*Fighting Depression*, by Harvey Ross, M.D., New York, Larchmont Books, 1975.

*Food, Teens and Behavior*, by Barbara Reed. Manitowoc, WI, Natural Press, 1983.

*Hypoglycemia: A Better Approach*, by Paavo Airola, Ph.D. Phoenix, Health Plus Publishers, 1977.

*Mind, Mood and Medicine: A Guide To The New Biopsychiatry*, by Paul H. Wender, M.D. and Donald F. Klein, M.D., NewYork, NAL, 1982.

*Psychodietetics*, by E. Cheraskin, M.D., D.M.D., William Ringsdorf Jr., D.M.D. with Arline Brecher. NewYork, Bantam Books, 1978.

*Sugar and Your Health*, by Ray C. Wunderlich, Jr., M.D. St. Petersburg, FL Good Health Publications, 1982.

*The Yeast Connection*, by William G. Crook, M.D., Jackson, Tenn., Professional Books, 1983.

*The Yeast Syndrome*, by John Parks Trowbridge, M.D. and Morton Walker, D.P.M., 1986.

# APPENDIX B

_____*Organizations That Supply Nutritional Information And Referral Lists*

Hypoglycemia Support Foundation, Inc., C/O Lifetime Books, Inc., 2131 Hollyvood Boulevard, #305, Hollywood, FL 33020.

Hypoglycemia Association, Inc. 18008 New Hampshire Ave., Box 165, Ashton, MD 20861

Academy of Orthomolecular Psychiatry, 1691 Northern Boulevard, Manhasset, Long Island, NewYork 11030.

Huxley Institute for Biosocial Research, Inc., 900 North Federal Highway, Boca Raton, FL 33432.

International Academy of Preventive Medicine, 34 Corporate Woods, Suite 469, 10950 Grandview, Overland Park, KS 66210.

International Academy of Applied Nutrition, P.O. Box 386 La Habra, CA 90631.

Nutrition For Optimal Health Association, Inc., P.O. Box 380, Winnetka, IL 60093.

Price Pottenger Nutritional Foundation, 5871 El Cajon, San Diego, CA 92115.

Society for Clinical Ecology, P.O. Box 16106, Denver, CO 80216.

American Holistic Medical Association, 4101 Lake Boone Trail, Suite 201, Raleigh, NC 27607

Association of Health Practitioners, P.O. Box 17990, Enrino, CA 91416-7990.

American Chiropractic Association, 1701 Clarendon Blvd., Arlington, VA 22209.

# APPENDIX C

## _____Bibliography

Abrahamson, E.M., M.D., and Pezet, A.W. *Body, Mind and Sugar*. NewYork, Avon Books, 1977.

Adams, Ruth, and Murray, Frank. *Is Low Blood Sugar Making You a Nutritional Cripple?* New York, Larchmont Press, 1970.

Airola, Paavo, Ph.D. *Hypoglycemia: A Better Approach*. Phoenix, Health Plus Publishers, 1977.

Anderson, Linnea, M.P.H., Dibble, Marjorie V., M.S., R.D., Turkki, Pirkko R., Ph.D., R.D., Mitchell, Helen S., Ph.D., Sc.D., Rynbergen, HenderikaJ., M.S. *Nutrition in Health and Disease, 17th Edition*. Philadelphia, J.B. Lippincott Company.

Appleton, Nancy, Ph.D. *Lick the Sugar Habit*. New York, Warner Books, Inc. 1986.

Atkinson, Holly, M.D. *Women and Fatigue.* NewYork, G.P. Putnam's Sons, 1985.

Bailey, Covert. *Fit or Fat?* Boston, Houghton Mifflin Company, 1977.

Bennion, Lynn J., M.D. *Hypoglycemia: Fact or Fad?* New York, Crown Publishers, Inc. 1983.

Bland, Jeffery, Ph.D. *Your Health Under Siege.* Vermont, The Stephen Greene Press, 1981.

Brennan, Dr. R.O. *Nutrigenetics.* NewYork, M. Evans and Company, 1975.

Budd, Martin L., N.D., D.O., Lic.Ac. *Low Blood Sugar.* New York, Sterling Publishing Co., Inc. 1981.

Cheraskin, E., M.D., D.M.D., William Ringsdorf, Jr., D.M.D. andJ.W. Clark, D.D.S., *Diet and Disease.* Connecticut, Keats Publishing, Inc. 1986.

Cheraskin E., M.D., D.M.D., Willaim Ringsdorf, Jr., D.M.D., with Arline Brecher. *Phychodietetics.* New York, Bantam Books, 1978.

Cheraskin, E., M.D., D.M.D., William Ringsdorf, Jr., D.M.D., and Emily L. Sisley, Ph.D. *The Vitamin C Connection.* NewYork, Harper & Row Publishers, Inc., 1983.

Crook, William G., M.D. *The Yeast Connection.* Tennessee, Professional Books, 1983.

Dufty, William. *Sugar Blues.* New York, Warner Books, Inc., 1975.

Fredericks, Carlton, Ph.D. *Carlton Fredericks' New Low Blood Sugar and You.* New York, Perigee Books, 1985.

Fredericks, Carlton, Ph.D. *Psycho-Nutrition*. NewYork, Grosset & Dunlap, 1976.

Krimmel, Patricia and Edward. *The Low Blood Sugar Hand book*. Bryn Mawr, PA, Franklin Publishers, 1984.

Lorenzani, Shirley, Ph.D. *Candida; A Twentieth Century Disease*. New Canaan, CT, Keats Publishing, Inc., 1986.

Martin, Clement G. *Low Blood Sugar; The Hidden Menace of Hypoglycemia*. New York, Arco Publishing Co., 1976.

*The Merck Manual of Diagnosis and Therapy, Twelfth Edition*. Rahway, NJ, Merck Sharp & Dohme Research Laboratories, Division of Merck & Co., Inc.

Milam, James R. and Katherine Ketcham, *Under the Influence*, New York, Bantam Books, 1981.

*Nutrition and Mental Health*. Hearing before the Select Committee on Nutrition and Human Needs of the United States Senate. California, Parker House, 1977.

Page, Melvin E., D.D.S., and H. Leon Abrams, Jr. *Your Body is Your Best Doctor*. New Canaan, CT, Keats Publishing, 1972.

Passwater, Richard A. *Supernutrition*. New York, Pocket Books, 1975

Pritikin, Nathan, with Patrick M. McGrady, Jr. *The Pritikin Program for Diet and Exercise*. New York, Grosset & Dunlap, 1979.

Rapp, Doris, J., M.D. *Allergies and the Hyperactive Child*. New York, Simon & Schuster, 1979.

Reed, Barbara. Foods, *Teens and Behavior*. Manitowoc, WI, Natural Press, 1983.

Ross, Harvey, M.D. *Fighting Depression*. NewYork, Larchmont Books, 1975.

Schauss, Alexander, *Diet, Crime and Delinquency*. Berkeley, CA, Parker House, 1981.

Saunders, Jeraldine, and Ross, Harvey, M.D. *Hypoglycemia: The Disease Your Doctor Won't Treat*, New York Pinnacle Press, 1980.

Smith, Lendon, M.D. *Feed Yourself Right*. New York, McGraw-Hill, 1983.

Smith, Lendon, M.D. *Foods For Healthy Kids*. New York, Berkley Books, 1981.

Truss, C. Orion, M.D. *The Missing Diagnosis*. Birmingham, The Missing Diagnosis, Inc., 1983.

Yudkin, John M.D. *Sweet and Dangerous*. New York, Bantam Books, 1972.

Weil, Andrew, M.D., and Rosen, Winifred. *Chocolate to Morphine*. Boston, Houghton Mifflin Co., 1983.

Weller, Charles. *How To Live With Hypoglycemia*. New York, Doubleday, 1968.

Wunderlich, Jr., Ray C., M.D. *Sugar and Your Health*. St Petersburg, FL, Good Health Publications, Johnny Reed, Inc., 1982.

Zack, Maura and Currier, Wilbur D., M.D. *Sugar Isn't Always Sweet*. Brea, CA, Uplift Books, 1983.